How to Survive (and Thrive) in a Toxic World

A User's Guide to Avoiding Chemicals for Radiant Health and a Clean Home Environment

Jeannette Russell

© 2009 Jeannette Russell

Cover picture courtesy of: Timeless Portraits by Liz

All Rights Reserved.

No part of this publication may be reproduced, stored in a retrieval system, or transmitted, in any form or by any means, electronic, mechanical, photocopying, recording, or otherwise, without the written permission of the author.

This edition published by
Dog Ear Publishing
4010 W. 86th Street, Ste H
Indianapolis, IN 46268

www.dogearpublishing.net

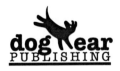

ISBN: 978-160844-118-1
This book is printed on acid-free paper.

Printed in the United States of America

I dedicate this book to our daughter, Brett Leigh Russell. She is still the most intelligent, courageous and loving soul we have ever encountered. We greatly look forward to being with her again. Your father and I will love you forever.

Disclaimer: The information provided is for educational purposes only. It is not meant to diagnose or treat any health condition and is not a replacement for treatment by a healthcare provider. If you are pregnant, nursing, taking medication, or have a medical condition, consult your physician before using the recommended products. These statements have not been evaluated by the Food and Drug Administration. The recommended products are not intended to diagnose, treat, cure, or prevent any disease. Jeannette Russell assumes no responsibility for the use or misuse of this material.

"If people let the government decide what foods they eat and what medicines they take, their bodies will soon be in as sorry a state as are the souls of those who live under tyranny."

-Thomas Jefferson

"The doctor of the future will give little medicine, but will interest his patients in the care of the human frame, diet, and in the cause and prevention of disease."

-Thomas Edison

Contents

Preface	ix
Why Should You Bother with this Book?	xi
How the Experts Have Failed Us	xiii
The Plan	xviii
Water	1
Why You Need to Filter Your Water	5
Water Fluoridation	11
USDA National Fluoride Data Base of Selected Foods and Beverages	19
Fluoride Calculator	40
Water Solutions	41
Your Food	47
The Art of Grocery Shopping	55
GMO Seeds and Food and their Danger to Humanity	63
Genetically Modified Ingredients Overview	67
Vitamins	75
Air	83
Air Solutions	85
Parents of Infants and Young Children	89
Vaccines	101
Vaccine Document for Your Pediatrician	107
How Cancer Cures Are Suppressed or Ignored By Pharmaceutical Corporations, Universities, Doctors, Government and Corporate Media	113

The Rewards of Change	117
Citizen Responsibility	119
Toxins of the Mind and Spirit	121
Brett's Story	123
Cancer Cured for Good	131

Preface

Sometimes, for some of us, a life event occurs that is so shattering, so incomprehensible, that we are forever transformed, almost overnight, into a different life lane, actually into a completely different person. This is what happened to me, and from this transformation has come this book.

In March 2001, our daughter, Brett Leigh Russell, was diagnosed with osteosarcoma, which is a deadly form of bone cancer, mostly occurring in children. This diagnosis stunned us, as our family had enjoyed good health for generations, and we thought we lived a "healthy" lifestyle. This started my quest to find out why such a dreadful disease had struck my child (and five other children in my county), and opened my eyes to information I had never known. The purpose of this book is to pass on this knowledge to you. My hope with this book is to transform the world. The old me would have "laughed" at my presumption and goal, but the new me says "of course" I can do this. I think every one of us has this potential. I truly believe that out of tragedy comes victory, if lessons learned are applied.

My motivation is a deep desire to help my fellow man. I believe it is the only reason for our existence on this planet, and by helping others I can transform myself.

Why Should You Bother with this Book?

After reading the preceding paragraphs, you might think "what does this have to do with me and my children?" Your financial health is at risk. I would like to make you aware of certain facts.

1. Most personal bankruptcies are caused by illness in the family
2. Childhood cancer is the number one cause of death in children except for accidents
3. Childhood cancer is increasing at an alarming rate (Brett's cancer, osteosarcoma, has increased FORTY PERCENT in just TEN YEARS!).
4. Cancer survival rates for people under 40 are unchanged from 20 years ago.

Despite my success in my career, I was forced to file for bankruptcy a year after Brett was diagnosed with cancer. I had excellent health insurance, however, when a child is diagnosed with cancer, it is impossible to go to work. Care is 24 hour shifts, runs to the hospital in the middle of the night, life and death decisions all the time. The bank that held the mortgage on my building that housed my business, exploited my situation and attempted to take away my property. The State and Federal government applied financial pressure and were also threatening us at the same time. Twenty years of hard work and everything I owned was at risk. So, while fighting for my daughter's life, I also had to deal with attacks from all sides. This was NOT FUN. At the hospital I watched children be dropped off AT THE CURB for chemo treatments, because their parents had to work. This is just one devastating aspect of this disease. There are other health issues that are serious, or not life threatening, that cost your family money, time, pain for your children, and prevents you from moving forward on your path to a great life. If you don't have at least two million dollars in the bank, YOU ARE AT RISK!

We always lived in the more affluent neighborhoods of Pittsburgh, Pennsylvania. Mothers mistakenly think that they are safe if they live in better places, BUT IT'S NOT TRUE. Your sense of security is a fantasy. There is no safe place. You must learn how to CREATE YOUR OWN SAFE ENVIRONMENT, and I can give you the information to do this. I will teach you what the real risks are and how to avoid them, begin to enjoy better health, and gain control of your life back from those entities that work every day to rob you of your birthright!

How the Experts Have Failed Us

Like most Americans, I thought that doctors and government officials, charged with protecting our health, had our best interests at heart. Starting in early March of 2001, the blinders started to come off as my thirteen year old daughter, Brett Leigh Russell, was diagnosed with a malignant bone tumor in her right leg. This is the catastrophic event I referred to in my preface. This one event put me on a life path a world away from the one I was living.

Ours is NOT the typical kid-gets-cancer story, because our family was not a typical family. My parents were immigrants from Italy. Our family had enjoyed incredible health most of our lives, for generations. We are a family of entrepreneurs and independent thinkers. Within a few months of each other, three family members were diagnosed with bone, ovarian and colon cancer, at ages thirteen, forty-one, and fifty-eight, respectively. We were like "WHAT THE HELL IS GOING ON"? I wanted to know WHY Brett had to fight for her life.

As I conducted my own extensive research to try to save my daughter's life, it became clear to me how misinformed we Americans really are, by our government and the corporations that have hijacked it. These corporations control every aspect of our lives, from doctors and hospitals to our food, water, and air. I specifically say "Americans" because the Europeans don't have as many problems in this area as we do. Their governments do a much better job of protecting their populations. Their regulations are more stringent, and more importantly, they are ENFORCED.

The purpose of this book is to inform you of the biggest hazards, of which you are probably unaware, as well as to give you solutions to protect yourself and your family. I took action to protect myself and my family over eight years ago and can testify that it is completely worthwhile to do so. Think of me as a modern insurance policy, which, if followed, will keep you and your family well, so that you can achieve your full potential in this life. Our current healthcare debate is a false one, because it doesn't address the real causes of poor health in America.

As much as I don't want to dwell on the past, I will interject past events, both personal and political, to make my points. It is a priceless gift from me to you, to ensure you will never endure the pain that we were forced to endure. During this process, while exposing the criminals who prey on your family's health for profit, I will give you a plan to stop them and regain control over your health and your prosperity. Let's face it, that without great health and prosperity, LIFE is a grim proposition.

Cleaning up your life and getting on the path of true health and independence is a process. One thing to remember is LITTLE CHANGES REALLY MATTER. It is the little things we expose ourselves to EVERY DAY that really determine our destiny and success in life. Never feel that the choice between a toxic product or a life enhancing product doesn't matter. It took me TWO YEARS to complete the change. It was gradual, affordable, and incredibly beneficial.

One thing you need to face when you get started is that you are in an undeclared WAR ZONE. It is YOU versus THE CORPORATIONS. They are systematically wrecking our health, as well as our country, and the FREEDOM we have treasured for over two hundred years, and it's TIME TO TAKE IT BACK. I will show you how to do it, because I have done it, and the rewards are great. I often hear that to do what I am proposing is too expensive, but I am here to tell you that IT WILL SAVE YOU MONEY. You have to understand that you will be transitioning from a QUANTITY lifestyle to a QUALITY lifestyle. It is truly a win/win type of situation. You SPEND LESS and FEEL BETTER. Some of the information (hell, maybe most of it) may be disturbing, but I'm hoping you will be adult, open your mind, forget the mass media propaganda, and LEARN THE TRUTH. Trust me, it's very cathartic!

My main concerns are your FOOD, WATER, and HOME ENVIRONMENT. As you gradually make changes in these areas, you will be surprised at how you start to feel. Hopefully you will be more calm, more energetic, less foggy, and more FEISTY. Always remember, IT IS REALLY EXPENSIVE TO BE SICK! It is completely avoidable. I speak as a financial survivor. At the time of my daughter's diagnosis, I was flying high. I was a successful wedding gown designer of twenty years. I had just purchased a commercial building in a prestigious neighborhood for our operations. My gowns were carried at Neiman Marcus. When a child gets cancer, you CANNOT work. While at the hospital, I would often help the kids that were there without their parents, because they HAD to work. They faired much more poorly because medical staff care is DEPLORABLE. Some of the things we endured during chemotherapy (for a mere $25,000 per session) were: a mattress so decrepit and slanted that my daughter had to hold onto the side rails to keep from falling on the floor; six and seven persons to a room (including family members of other patients) who snored, used my shampoo and shared my daughter's bathroom, despite the terrible risk of infection; regularly incorrectly prescribed medicines; and student doctors when my daughter was at death's door. Not bad for over a million dollars, right? However, we were talking about money. The question begs asking: What if tomorrow you lost your main source of income, and were unable to replace it in any fashion? How long would it be before you were in BIG TROUBLE? I lost millions of dollars and a great career, despite the fact that I had GREAT health insurance. My only wish at that time, was that I wish I had had more to lose. The small changes you will be making will save you MILLIONS in the long run, and aren't we all interested in a long run? I don't often hear from people that they don't want to live very long, and when it is time to go, they hope it will be very painful as well as bankrupt them! Yeah, it's worth it to change.

My goal isn't to frighten you, it's to get you thinking seriously about changing how you think and spend your money. Your purchasing habits can be a weapon in your war against the corporations OR it can be the weapon the corporations use AGAINST you, to pull you ever deeper into dependence upon them. I am a Patrick Henry kind of American "GIVE ME LIBERTY OR GIVE ME DEATH!" I really love that guy! He brings tears to my eyes. I'll be right back with THE PLAN.

The Plan

My plan is pretty straightforward. I am going to show you where the real risks are, in your lifestyle and home, and direct you to solutions. The discussion is about your AIR, your WATER, your FOOD and your ENVIRONMENT. The things you interact with on a daily basis determine your destiny. When you are in charge of these things, you are calling the shots in your life. This is what has been slowly stolen from us by our government and the corporations that control them for the last fifty years. It is past time to redeem our control over our own bodies and lives. Let's proceed....

Water

Clean water is ESSENTIAL to life. Good health is IMPOSSIBLE without CLEAN water. Here are some facts about water and YOU:

1. About 83% of our bodies consist of water.
2. Our brains consists of about 70% water.
3. Our lungs are about 90% water.
4. Water helps digest our food, transport waste, and control body temperature.
5. Pure water has a neutral pH of 7.
6. Water is UNIQUE. It is the ONLY substance on earth found in all three states, liquid, solid, and gas.
7. ONE drop of OIL can render 25 litres of water unfit for drinking.
8. Health problems related to water pollution, in general, are estimated to cost ALL of us MILLIONS per year.
9. It is recommended that we drink about 8 glasses of fluid (preferably water) everyday.
10. About 70% of the earth's surface is water. Fresh water lakes and rivers, ice, snow, and underwater aquifers hold 2.5% of the world's water. 68.9% of earth's fresh water exists in the form of glaciers and permanent snow cover. (You know, the ones that are melting. The climate change deniers say "Don't worry your pretty little head about this!")

NOTES

I know it can be boring to read facts, but THESE facts are important. It can be surmised, using your common sense, that it is vital to your health to drink CLEAN water. If you drink unpurified water, you can expect to be sick with either acute illness (poisoning) or chronic illness (cancer, diabetes, or heart disease). NOT FUN!!! It is very stupid to WASTE water and/or POLLUTE water. The quality of your body and blood is determined by the QUALITY of your water.

So remember these equations:

Dirty water = POOR health

Clean water = RADIANT health

NOTES

Why You Need to Filter Your Water

An environmental group conducted a study in 42 states of thousands of water authorities. They found 141 unregulated chemicals, which the EPA has never even established safe levels, and another 119 regulated chemicals that were found in a two and a half year analysis. The top ten states with the most contaminated water were: California, Wisconsin, Arizona, Florida, North Carolina, Pennsylvania (my state), Texas, New York, Nevada, and Illinois. I hope you are upset about this, and sadly, there is more to come. I am trying REALLY HARD to make you mad! REALLY MAD! How can the government allow corporations to poison a resource so VITAL to our existence? They have obviously betrayed our trust, and until we straighten this out and make them DO THE JOBS FOR WHICH THEY ARE PAID, I again recommend you filter your water as much as possible. The good news is that there are many products available now to help you protect you and your family's health. Many people don't realize that 70% of the water you absorb everyday is from your SHOWER. This is the easiest to remedy. There are many shower filters available online. I will have a list of recommendations to help you make these changes at the end of this section.

Just a personal anecdote here: when I had traveled to Germany for treatment for my daughter, we realized how much cleaner their water was, than ours. My hair only needed washing every other day. It was the first time in YEARS that I required a shower cap! Of course this saves on shampoo and

NOTES

conditioner. As I promised, you will see that living 'green' also saves you money.

Regarding water for drinking and cooking, of course it is important to clean up this area as well. I mentioned the shower first because it has the largest impact and a shower filter will get you feeling better fast. I don't recommend taking baths until you are at the point of getting ALL of the water in your home cleaned up. I will discuss this at the end of this chapter. I am trying to give options to everyone, regardless of their income. The most expensive systems are the POINT OF ENTRY systems that clean all the water in your house. I will present all of the alternatives and you can decide what you can afford. Remember that ANY change you make is GOOD. Don't feel that if you have to ease into this process, that small steps won't help you, because it's not true. The less you burden your liver, kidneys, skin, and lymph (your detoxification systems), the more they can help you stay well!

I HATE BOTTLED WATER! It is so bad for your health and a pox on the planet. I beg you, BUY A REUSEABLE WATER BOTTLE. It saves you a lot of money, reduces trash and gives you water you KNOW about. I believe in the DEVIL YOU KNOW. Your local tap water is water you can become familiar with, but who knows what is in your bottle of water. This is an UNREGULATED INDUSTRY. It is on the HONOR system! What a hoot. There IS NO HONOR IN THESE CORPORATIONS. They will only do the bare minimum to stay operating, and not a PENNY more. There are only a few reusable water bottles that I will recommend. It is very important that you get a bottle that won't leach anything into your water, so be very picky about your bottle and make sure your bottle is CLEAN. Check the recommended cleaning for your bottle and make sure it is something you can live with. Remember that the minutes you devote every day to protecting your health, prevent you from spending endless hours in a doctor's waiting room or a hospital room. These are BAD places to AVOID at all costs. Your reward will be a great life of freedom to live your life. It is worth a few min-

NOTES

utes everyday. Well it is time to tackle an issue that I dread talking about, BUT I HAVE TO TALK ABOUT IT. It is so important that it will receive its own chapter. Please keep an open mind and listen to the FACTS, not the propaganda we have been fed for over 60 years. OK.....

NOTES

Water Fluoridation

Eight years ago, I was like everybody else in America. I thought WATER FLUORIDATION WAS A GOOD THING! I bought fluoridated tooth paste, I made sure that Brett got regular fluoride treatments at the dentist. If I bought bottled water, I would gravitate toward the ones with advertised fluoride. I mean, there was NO WAY my government, The American Dental Association and my dentist would lie to me, right? Well the right answer to that comment would be YES THEY WOULD! I don't know if you can imagine how I felt, when I was researching my daughter's disease (bone cancer), that fluoride was a factor in her disease? This was a very low moment for me. I felt HORRIBLE. I actually had been subjecting her to a chemical that was contributing to her disease. The scientific evidence AGAINST fluoridation is very strong. It was strong enough for most of Europe to BAN water fluoridation OVER A DECADE AGO! SO WHAT THE HELL IS GOING ON IN OUR COUNTRY? Are American bodies made differently from European bodies? Do we have some sort of SPECIAL PROTECTION that they don't? Of course we don't. We just have more powerful corporation lobbies that can bribe our government officials and allow this deadly chemical in our water, food, and environment. Thanks Republicans! Thanks Democrats! They are equal opportunity sell outs. I know we are all complaining about our leaders (what a joke) these days, but actually they have been dreadful for at least 60 years. A fantastic book has been written by Christopher Bryson called "The Fluoride Deception". It discloses how this terrible betrayal of the public health came about, the criminals who expedited it, as

NOTES

well as the consequences from putting this toxin in our water. I am just going to lay out a few FACTS about fluoride that the average person doesn't know, but NEEDS to know:

1. Fluoride makes very poor quality bone. There is a much higher rate of hip fractures in communities that fluoridate their water than those who don't. So if you have suffered a hip fracture, you certainly want to stop ingesting fluoride as much as possible.
2. Fluoride is harmful to your thyroid. The thyroid is a very important gland and a myriad of health problems can be caused by a malfunctioning thyroid.
3. The fluoride used by water authorities in your water is a waste product of the pesticide industry. It is industrial waste, not the sodium fluoride on the periodic chart you studied in school. Water fluoridation is an ENORMOUS help to industry, because many industries GET PAID for an industrial WASTE PRODUCT.
4. The EPA stipulates that the fluoride waste products they produce MUST BE DISPOSED OF IN THE SAME MANNER AS NUCLEAR WASTE. Doesn't that blow your mind? The fluoride added to your water is as dangerous as NUCLEAR WASTE! That really makes me want to guzzle down that water!
5. The CDC has (FINALLY) stated that mothers with newborns SHOULD NOT USE TAP WATER TO MAKE FORMULA BECAUSE IT WILL LOWER A BABY'S I.Q. That's because fluoride is a neurotoxin. You know, brain poison (besides being rat poison as well). How disgusted are you at this point?
6. The National Kidney Foundation has also, belatedly, discovered their balls, and has ALSO warned those who use dialysis to NOT USE

NOTES

FLUORIDATED WATER FOR THEIR TREATMENTS AS THEY COULD DIE! I guess that it was this kind of information that persuaded Europe to abandon this practice, yet here they STILL PROMOTE IT!

7. The latest Harvard research AGAIN shows that there are 40% more bone tumors in children who live in fluoridated neighborhoods than those that don't fluoridate. These same statistics were discovered when comparing Ireland, which still fluoridates, and Northern Ireland, which does not, that Ireland had 40% more bone tumors than their northern relatives.

8. The EPA states that 1ppm of fluorides is "safe" for the general public. They obviously feel that more than that is harmful, right? Well, we are ALL getting way too much fluoride because IT IS IN EVERY FOOD PRODUCT MADE WITH TAP WATER. The USDA has recently published a study of over 400 foods and their fluoride content. I will be publishing this list, and then you will be able to compute just how much fluoride you and your family are eating. This will enable you to AVOID those foods that have unsafe amounts of this toxin. I will be getting into this much more in my FOOD section.

9. Fluoride is a main ingredient in medications for depression (even though it causes depression!). I believe future generations are going to shake their heads when they learn what we did to ourselves.

10. There is NO difference in the number of cavities of children in fluoridated communities, as opposed to non-fluoridated communities. Good dental health is a NUTRITION issue and a MAINTENANCE issue. I will also have some tips about dental health as well.

NOTES

This is just a small amount of information on the harm caused by fluoride. The book I referred to earlier is an eye-opening read about the duplicity of corporations, of our government, and as well as the compliant medical establishment. You know, THE EXPERTS WE TRUST TO LOOK OUT FOR US. It's a sad joke. We're on our own, baby. It's time to take back your health from these parasites. I am going to make it easier for you to regain your health and your independence.

NOTES

2004 USDA National Fluoride Database of Selected Beverages and Foods

Intended goal of fluoridation: Delivery of **1 milligram of fluoride per day**
1 milligram/liter = 1ppm (parts per million)

Food Group	Item	Mean mcg/100g **
	Baby Foods:	
	Cereal, mixed, with applesauce and bananas, junior	1
	Cereal, oatmeal, with applesauce and bananas, junior	8
	Cereal, rice, with applesauce and bananas, strained	16
	Cereal, rice, with mixed fruit, junior	3
	Dessert, custard pudding, vanilla, junior	4
	Dessert, Dutch apple, junior	2
	Dessert, fruit dessert, junior	18
	Dessert, peach cobbler, junior	8
	Dinner, chicken noodle, junior	29
	Dinner, macaroni and cheese, junior	6
	Dinner, spaghetti, tomato, meat, junior	2
	Dinner, turkey and rice, junior	20
	Dinner, vegetables and beef, junior	21
	Dinner, vegetables and ham, junior	14
	Dinner, vegetables and turkey, junior	8
	Fruit, apple and blueberry, junior	1
	Fruit, applesauce, junior	2

NOTES

USDA National Flouride Data Base

Fruit, applesauce, strained	1
Fruit, apricot with tapioca, junior	0
Fruit, bananas, pineapple with tapioca, junior	16
Fruit, bananas with tapioca, junior	36
Fruit, mango with tapioca, strained	12
Fruit, peaches with sugar, strained	0
Fruit, peaches, junior	3
Fruit, pears and pineapple, junior	1
Fruit, pears, junior	9
Fruit, pears, strained	1
Fruit, plums with tapioca, junior	34
Fruit, prunes, without Vitamin C, strained	2
Juice, apple	12
Juice, apple and cherry	67
Juice, apple and grape	45
Juice, apple and peach	19
Juice, apple and prune	13
Juice, apple-cranberry	10
Meat, beef, junior	2
Meat, ham, junior	3
Meat, lamb, junior	10
Meat, turkey, junior	44
Vegetables and bacon, junior	3
Vegetables, carrots, strained	1
Vegetables, carrots, junior	12
Vegetables, corn, creamed, junior	32
Vegetables, green beans, junior	12
Vegetables, green beans, strained	16
Vegetables, peas, strained	25
Vegetables, squash, junior	5
Vegetables, squash, strained	1
Vegetables, sweet potatoes, junior	10
Vegetables, sweet potatoes, strained	1
Baked products:	
Biscuits, refrigerated dough, baked	26
Bread, all (white and whole wheat)	39
Bread, rye	51
Bread stuffing, prepared, baked	51
Brownie, with nuts	38
Cake, all	22
Cookies, without raisins, all	16
Cookies, oatmeal raisin	69
Cornbread	11
Crackers, all	24
Doughnuts	30
Éclair, chocolate	13
Muffin, blueberry	39
Pancakes, buttermilk, frozen	20

NOTES

USDA National Flouride Data Base

Pie, apple, frozen, heated	13
Pie, pumpkin, frozen, heated	32
Rolls, hamburger and hot dog	25
Snack type, cake roll	49
Snack type, chocolate cup cake, cream filled	38
Snack type, oatmeal cream pie	41
Tortillas, flour	33
Waffles, frozen, KELLOGG'S EGGO	35
Beef products:	
Beef, cooked and raw	22
Beef, liver, pan cooked with added fat	5
Beverages:	
Alcoholic beverage, beer, light	45
Alcoholic beverage, beer, regular	44
Alcoholic beverage, distilled, all (gin, rum, vodka, whiskey), 80 proof	9
Alcoholic beverage, wine, red	105
Alcoholic beverage, wine, white	202
Carbonated, cola, diet, fast food type, without ice	78
Carbonated, cola, fast food type, without ice	65
Carbonated, cola, PEPSI, all regions	32
Carbonated, cola, PEPSI, Mid-West	36
Carbonated, cola, PEPSI, Northeast	27
Carbonated, cola, PEPSI, South	45
Carbonated, cola, PEPSI, West	13
Carbonated, cola, COCA-COLA, all regions	49
Carbonated, cola, COCA-COLA, Mid-West	46
Carbonated, cola, COCA-COLA, Northeast	53
Carbonated, cola, COCA-COLA, South	57
Carbonated, cola, COCA-COLA, West	36
Carbonated, cola, DIET PEPSI, all regions	48
Carbonated, cola, DIET PEPSI, Mid-West	46
Carbonated, cola, DIET PEPSI, Northeast	46
Carbonated, cola, DIET PEPSI, South	66
Carbonated, cola, DIET PEPSI, West	25
Carbonated, cola, DIET COKE, all regions	60
Carbonated, cola, DIET COKE, Mid-West	69
Carbonated, cola, DIET COKE, Northeast	58
Carbonated, cola, DIET COKE, South	72
Carbonated, cola, DIET COKE, West	33
Carbonated, cola, PEPSI ONE, all regions	40
Carbonated, cola, PEPSI ONE, Mid-West	47
Carbonated, cola, PEPSI ONE, Northeast	31
Carbonated, cola, PEPSI ONE, South	56
Carbonated, cola, PEPSI ONE, West	18
Carbonated, ginger ale	80
Carbonated, grape soda	93

NOTES

Carbonated, lemon-lime, fast food type, without ice	64
Carbonated, lemon-lime, SPRITE, all regions	48
Carbonated, lemon-lime, SPRITE, Mid-West	47
Carbonated, lemon-lime, SPRITE, Northeast	48
Carbonated, lemon-lime, SPRITE, South	59
Carbonated, lemon-lime, SPRITE, West	29
Carbonated, orange soda	84
Carbonated, root beer	83
Carbonated, water, fruit-flavored	105
Chocolate-flavor beverage, mix for milk, powder	5
Coffee, brewed	91
Cranberry juice cocktail and blends, light, ready-to-drink	70
Fruit drink, CAPRI-SUN, ready-to-drink	71
Fruit drink, HAWAIIAN PUNCH, ready-to-drink	44
Fruit drink, HI-C, ready-to-drink	22
Fruit drink, MINUTE MAID punch, ready-to-drink	17
Fruit drink, other brands, ready-to-drink	54
Fruit flavored drinks, prepared from powder	42
Fruit flavored drinks, KOOL-AID, ready-to-drink	43
Fruit flavored drink, SUNNY DELIGHT, ready-to-drink	68
Fruit juice drink, apple, ready-to-drink	104
Fruit juice drink, blends (not cranberry), ready-to-drink	49
Fruit juice drink, FIVE ALIVE, ready-to-drink	8
Fruit juice drink, grape, ready-to-drink	32
Fruit juice drink, orange, ready-to-drink	55
Lemonade, ready to drink	25
Tea, brewed, microwave, all	*322
Tea, brewed, microwave, Mid-West	*319
Tea, brewed, microwave, Northeast	*309
Tea, brewed, microwave, South	*322
Tea, brewed, microwave, West	*310
Tea, brewed, decaffeinated, all	*269
Tea, brewed, decaffeinated, Mid-West	*293
Tea, brewed, decaffeinated, Northeast	*279
Tea, brewed, decaffeinated, South	*264
Tea, brewed, decaffeinated, West	*247
Tea, brewed, regular, all	*373
Tea, brewed, regular, Mid-West	*393
Tea, brewed, regular, Northeast	*357
Tea, brewed, regular, South	*381
Tea, brewed, regular, West	*355
Tea, iced, ARIZONA, ready-to-drink	123
Tea, iced, COOL NESTEA Natural Lemon, ready-to-drink	90
Tea, iced, LIPTON BRISK Lemon, ready-to-drink	72
Tea, instant, powder, unsweetened	89772
Tea, instant, powder, unsweetened, prepared with tap water	335

NOTES

USDA Flouride Data Base

Tea, instant, powder, with lemon and sugar	584
Tea, instant, powder, with lemon and sugar, prepared with tap water	116
Thirst quencher (sport drink), GATORADE, ready-to-drink	34
Thirst quencher (sport drink), POWERADE, ready-to-drink	62
Water, bottled, AQUAFINA	5
Water, bottled, CALISTOGA	7
Water, bottled, CRYSTAL GEYSER	24
Water, bottled, DANNON	11
Water, bottled, DANNON FLUORIDE TO GO	78
Water, bottled, DASANI	7
Water, bottled, EVIAN	10
Water, bottled, NAYA	14
Water, bottled, PERRIER	31
Water, bottled, POLAND SPRINGS	10
Water, bottled, PROPEL FITNESS WATER	2
Water, bottled, SARATOGA	20
Water, bottled, VERYFINE FRUIT2O Water	6
Water, bottled, VOLVIC	34
Water, bottled, store brand	16
Water, frozen (ice)	11
Waters, tap, all regions, all (includes municipal and well)	71
Waters, tap, all regions, municipal $	81
Waters, tap, all regions, well	26
Waters, tap, Mid-West, all (includes municipal and well)	88
Waters, tap, Mid-West, municipal	99
Waters, tap, Mid-West, well	53
Waters, tap, Northeast, all (includes municipal and well)	69
Waters, tap, Northeast, municipal	74
Waters, tap, Northeast, well	9
Waters, tap, South, all (includes municipal and well)	76
Waters, tap, South, municipal	93
Waters, tap, South, well	10
Waters, tap, West, all (includes municipal and well)	47
Waters, tap, West, municipal	51
Waters, tap, West, well	24
Breakfast cereals:	
Corn flakes	17
Farina, enriched, cooked	51
Granola, with raisins	33
Grits, cooked	56
Oatmeal, cooked	72
Oatmeal, instant, flavored, prepared	50
Oat rings	50
Presweetened, ready-to-eat	24
Raisin bran	65

NOTES

Rice, ready-to-eat	17
Rice and corn, lightly sweetened, ready-to-eat	31
Wheat, ready-to-eat	27
Cereal grains and pastas:	
Macaroni and spaghetti, cooked	7
Macaroni and spaghetti, uncooked	18
Noodles, egg, cooked	6
Rice, cooked	41
Dairy and egg products:	
Butter	3
Buttermilk	4
Cheese, American, processed	35
Cheese, cheddar	35
Cheese, cottage	32
Cream, fluid, half and half	3
Cream substitute, powdered	112
Egg, cooked	5
Egg, raw	1
Milk, chocolate	5
Milk, evaporated	8
Milk, 1%	3
Milk, 2%	3
Milk, skim	3
Yogurt, fruit, strawberry	9
Yogurt, plain, low-fat	12
Fast foods:	
Chicken McNUGGETS, McDONALD'S	16
Coleslaw	11
Dessert, DAIRY QUEEN, BLIZZARD	13
Dessert, WENDY'S, FROSTY	19
French fries, McDONALD'S	115
Hamburger on roll, quarter pound patty, with condiments	28
Pizza	31
Shake	14
Steak and cheese sandwich	37
Fats and oils:	
Mayonnaise	9
Margarine	5
Margarine-like spread	25
Salad dressing, mayonnaise type	4
Salad dressings	27
Vegetable oil, corn	1
Finfish and shellfish products:	
Crab, canned	210
Fish, cooked (includes broiled and fried)	18

NOTES

USDA National Flouride Data Base

Fish sticks, baked	134
Shrimp, canned	201
Shrimp, fried	166
Tuna, light, canned in water	19
Tuna, canned in oil, drained	31
Fruits and fruit products:	
Apple juice, DOLE, ready-to-drink	58
Apple juice, JUICY JUICE, ready-to-drink	48
Apple juice, MINUTE MAID, ready-to-drink	28
Apple juice, MOTT'S, ready-to-drink	28
Apple, raw, with peel	3
Applesauce, sweetened	5
Avocado, raw	7
Bananas, raw	2
Cantaloupe, raw	1
Cherries, sweet, raw	2
Cranberry sauce	2
Fruit cocktail, canned	9
Grapefruit, raw	1
Grapefruit juice	45
Grape juice blend (apple and grape), JUICY JUICE, ready-to-drink	102
Grape juice blend (apple, grape and pear), MINUTE MAID, ready-to-drink	43
Grape juice blend (apple and grape), MOTT'S, ready-to-drink	27
Grape juice, WELCH'S, ready-to-drink	72
Grape juice, white	204
Grapes, raw	49
Nectar, fruit	12
Orange, juice, frozen, concentrate	20
Orange, juice, frozen, concentrate, prepared with tap water	58
Orange juice, DEAN, ready-to-drink	52
Orange juice, MINUTE MAID, ready-to-drink	31
Peaches, canned	7
Peaches, raw	4
Pears, raw	2
Pears, canned	8
Pineapple, canned, juice pack	2
Pineapple juice, canned	6
Plums, dried (prunes), uncooked	4
Plums, purple, raw	2
Prune juice	60
Raisins	234
Strawberries, raw	4

NOTES

Watermelon, raw	1
Lamb, veal and game:	
Lamb chop, pan cooked with added fat	32
Veal cutlet, breaded, pan cooked with added fat	21
Veal, liver, pan cooked with added fat	5
Legumes and legume products:	
Beans, baked, canned, with pork	54
Beans, mature, boiled	2
Cowpeas common (black eyes), boiled	3
Peanut butter, creamy	3
Peanuts, dry roasted, salted	16
Meals, entrees and side dishes:	
Beef stew	57
Casserole, beef, tomato and pasta	67
Chicken potpie	75
Chicken and noodle casserole, homemade	16
Chili con carne, beef and beans, canned	45
Frozen meal, fried chicken, mashed potatoes, cornbread, and/or vegetable	48
Lasagna, homemade	18
Macaroni and cheese, prepared from mix	33
Mashed potato and gravy	84
Meatloaf	30
Spaghetti, with meat sauce	38
Spaghetti, with sauce, no meat, canned	24
Ravioli, CHEF BOYARDEE, beef, with meat sauce, canned	13
Turkey, broccoli, cheese bake	28
Turkey potpie	166
Nut and seed products:	
Pecans, packaged, unsalted	10
Pork products:	
Bacon, cooked	22
Bacon, raw	4
Ham, cured, baked	20
Pork, chop, baked	38
Pork, chop, pan cooked, with added fat	129
Pork, roast, cooked	42
Poultry products:	
Chicken, cooked (includes fried and roasted)	15
Turkey, roast	21
Sausages and luncheon meats:	
Bologna	29
Ham and cheese loaf	36
Hot dogs, beef	48
Sausage, pork	18

NOTES

USDA National Flouride Data Base

Sausage (includes salami, not hard)	41
Snacks:	
Chips, corn and tortilla	50
Popcorn, oil popped	6
Potato chip	65
Potato chip, baked	106
Soups, sauces, and gravies:	
Sauce, cheese	29
Sauce, spaghetti, canned	37
Sauce, tartar	30
Sauce, white	4
Gravy, beef	99
Gravy, brown, prepared from mix	57
Soup, beef bouillon, canned, reconstituted	29
Soup, chicken broth	61
Soup, chicken noodle, canned, reconstituted	35
Soup, clam chowder	36
Soup, corn chowder	132
Soup, minestrone	86
Soup, pea	76
Soup, tomato, canned reconstituted, with milk	7
Soup, vegetable beef, canned, reconstituted	43
Spices and herbs:	
Pepper, black	34
Salt, iodized	2
Sweets:	
Candies, caramels	27
Candies, milk chocolate	5
Candies, M&M MARS, "M&M's" Milk Chocolate Candies	17
Candies, REESE'S Peanut Butter Cups	9
Candies, M&M MARS, SNICKERS Bar	36
Gum	5
Frozen novelties, ice type, regular, all flavors	74
Frozen novelties, ice type, sugar free, all flavors	89
Frozen novelties, juice type	77
Frozen novelties, ice cream sandwich	27
Frozen yogurts, chocolate	40
Frozen yogurts, vanilla	26
Gelatin desserts, strawberry, prepared	69
Honey, bottled	7
Jam, strawberry	19
Jellies	73
Ice creams, chocolate	23
Ice creams, vanilla	15
Bread pudding	74
Puddings, instant, prepared with whole milk	22

NOTES

USDA National Flouride Data Base

Sugar, granulated	1
Syrup, pancake	44
Vegetables and vegetable products:	
Asparagus, cooked	22
Beans, snap (includes cooked, canned, frozen)	19
Beets, canned	26
Broccoli, boiled	4
Cabbage, boiled	1
Carrots, cooked	47
Carrots, raw	3
Catsup	12
Cauliflower, boiled	1
Celery, raw	4
Coleslaw	10
Collard greens, boiled	27
Corn, frozen, kernels cut off cob, unprepared	15
Corn, canned	18
Corn, cream style, canned	28
Cucumber, raw	1
Lettuce	5
Lima beans, immature seeds, frozen, boiled	7
Mixed vegetables, canned	37
Mushrooms, canned	10
Onion rings, breaded, fried, frozen, heated	55
Onions, raw	1
Peas, green (includes cooked and canned)	29
Peppers, sweet, green, raw	2
Pickles, cucumber, dill	24
Potatoes, boiled	49
Potatoes, french fried, frozen, heated	26
Potatoes, hashed brown	44
Potatoes, mashed	39
Potatoes, puffs, frozen, prepared	6
Potatoes, russet, baked	45
Potatoes, scalloped	31
Radishes, raw	6
Sauerkraut, canned	7
Spinach, cooked	38
Squash, cooked (includes summer and winter)	2
Sweet potatoes	14
Sweet potatoes, candied, home prepared	8
Tomatoes, canned	6
Tomatoes, raw	2
Tomato juice, canned	7

NOTES

Tomato sauce, canned	35
Tossed salad	5

**mcg/100g = ppm * 100 (beverages corrected for specific gravity)

* indicates fluoride is intensified by heating. This applies to water, as well.

Daily Fluoride Calculator

Menu	Glasses of Water	Drinks	Showers/Baths	Toothpaste	Alcoholic Drinks
Breakfast					
Lunch					
Dinner					
Snacks					

Water Solutions

Affordable options:

1. Stop buying bottled water. It's expensive and the quality is uncertain. Bottled water is UNREGULATED. Buy a stainless steel water bottle and USE it! One good company that has high quality stainless steel inside the bottle is EARTHLUST at www.earthlust.com.
2. Get a shower filter. You may be surprised that I am giving this tip a higher priority than what you are drinking at home. The reason is that about seventy percent of the toxins that get into your system penetrate through your skin during your daily shower. Remember that it is the things that you do EVERY DAY that will determine your health. All of the chemicals in your water, like chlorine, arsenic and a host of others, hurt your lungs, your liver, and kidneys, as well as harming your beauty attributes like your hair and skin. So a shower filter will help protect your insides AND your outside! A few suggestions are available at www.equinoxproducts.com. You will become familiar with this site, as I really like and use their products. They are very well priced and effective. They offer a shower filter for under fifty dollars. It lasts TWO YEARS and requires no interim filters during the following two years. There are other filters that may be less expensive, but you have to change the filters every few

NOTES

months. So when you are purchasing a filter, make sure you add on the extra filters you will need to buy and install. Look at the TOTAL cost of the filter over two years.

Ultimate solution:

This is where I have ended up today concerning water filtration in my own home. All of the steps I have outlined above are measures I have used when money was scarce. I have "graduated" to the system I use now, as my income stabilized. It is called a Point of Entry system. It is whole house filtration that cleans ALL of the water that enters your home. It is installed next to your water meter or at the place where water is piped into your home. It consists of three parts. There is a sediment filter, then a fluoride filter, and finally a tank that removes all other contaminants. This is where you need to be headed, ultimately. This type of filter means that you can shower and bathe in clean water. You can cook and drink with clean water. Your portable water bottle will have clean water. You will be stunned with the health benefits. Clean water keeps your God-given machine humming along, enabling you to accomplish your goals and achieve your destiny with energy and peace. This is a priceless gift today. I purchased my system from www.equinoxproducts.com. It cost fifteen hundred dollars with an additional Two hundred fifty for installation using a registered plumber. If you are handy, you can avoid this added cost. The sediment filter needs to be changed every one to three months depending upon the water that runs through it. Our water is so impure that we have to change it every month. These filters cost four dollars each. The other tanks will last about seven years. I love this system and I love my water. It is delicious and feels great. Unlike reverse osmosis, there is no water waste. This company makes its own filters and sells them directly to the public, so it is the best price for whole house water filters. Other systems that I have researched were between five thousand and ten thousand

NOTES

dollars. I am happy to know that deadly fluoride is no longer undermining my health. Also, my pipes will last longer because fluoride can no longer corrode the seams in my pipes and release lead into my water. I would recommend starting with this system, if you have the seventeen hundred and fifty dollars to do it, or if you can not right now, have it as an ultimate goal.

Equinox Products have many options for kitchen and bath on their website. Any action that you take will help to ease the toxic burden on your body. Do whatever you can afford and be happy about it. I will repeat my mantra:

SMALL CHANGES MATTER!

NOTES

Your Food

It is no accident that I titled this section "YOUR" food. Once you eat something, it becomes a part of you. It can be something that enhances your body, or harms it. Shortly after Brett was diagnosed and about two weeks into my research, I switched to organic food. I made a drastic change because our situation was life or death. The purpose of this book is to prevent what happened to us, from happening to you. Your story doesn't, and mustn't, be our story. Believe me when I say "you never want to be us!" The quality of your blood and organs is dependent upon what you use to build them. Again, trust your common sense to lead you in a good direction. You don't require a scientist, doctor, nutritionist, head of FDA, AMA, ADA, CDC, or any other initials to validate what your common sense can see so plainly.

Another simple equation:

DIRTY FOOD= DIRTY BODY and

POOR QUALITY FOOD = POOR QUALITY

BLOOD AND ORGANS.

Think back now and tell me how many minutes have you discussed food with your doctor…..Have you EVER had this conversation? Tragically, not many people do. I can't decide what is worse, the no conversation or the conversation with bad information. I have spoken to many doctors and nutritionists, and most of them JUST DON'T GET IT. They

NOTES

don't think vitamins are necessary, organic food is a waste of money, etcetera. Nutritionists are taught NOTHING about real nutrition. In America, people would be HORRIFIED to put tainted gas or oil in their cars, but will fill themselves with JUNK. Our bodies are INCREDIBLE machines that deserve RESPECT (at least as much respect as our cars!) We have physically evolved over MILLIONS of years. Our hands alone are small miracles. Our brains are so complicated we STILL don't know hardly ANYTHING about them. We are walking, talking miracles that house amazing souls, part of an amazing Universe. Take a moment and give thanks for this miraculous machine that has been given to you, to use to expand your soul. It deserves, at the very least, as much attention as your car! THANKS GOD!

Again, I'm going to give you some facts about conventional food that you may not know:

1. Conventional foods grown by BIG AGRIBUSINESS contain FORTY PERCENT less nutrients than organic food. A local magazine in our area had an article by a local doctor who loudly proclaimed there is NO DIFFERENCE between conventional and organic food. OOPS! She is just another expert failing her patients and the public. So really, conventional food isn't much of a bargain, is it?
2. The pesticides used ON and IN our food not only harm insects and animals, they harm US. They pollute our bodies, our water, our air and our soil, and they are not necessary.
3. Conventional food is cheaper than organic food. This IS NOT TRUE if you look at the medical costs involved from being sick because you are POISONED, or denied necessary nutrients. Eating conventional foods is SLOW poisoning.
4. GMO foods are downright SCARY! This experiment, by Big corporations like MONSAN-

NOTES

TO, on us is a criminal activity, in my opinion. Slowly, the truth about this criminal activity is coming out. The research so far is very bad. Health problems that are implicated by current scientific research are infertility (who needs a condom?), allergies, cancer, liver disorders, immune dysfunction, animal deaths, and GMO that persist in the human gut. To date, 183 Indian farmers have committed suicide. These dangerous games the insane people at Monsanto are playing PUTS OUR ENTIRE FOOD SYSTEM AT RISK. It appears that their ultimate goal is to hold our food hostage, much the same as Middle East OIL, and we all know how well THAT is going! The USDA should be held in CRIMINAL CONTEMPT for allowing these corporations to compromise our very survival. If you eat conventional foods, you CANNOT AVOID THESE GMO ingredients. In our section titled Sources of GMO ingredients, you can become informed about what is really in your food, as the USDA refuses to signify GMO ingredients. GMOs deserve their own chapter.

5. Laura Bush was ADAMANT that the First Family only be fed ORGANIC FOOD. While she was being ADAMANT, her husband was out promoting GMO foods for all of us "little people". Thanks again George, for undermining your citizens in yet another way. He linked purchasing GMO seed to Aid for Africa. No GMO seed, no AID. Yeah, he was a real peach. Obama and his family are also eating organic. As I said, the hypocrisy is bipartisan.

6. Processed food, whether organic or conventional should be a small part of your diet. Simply, this is food in boxes.

NOTES

7. Many countries in Europe have banned EIGHT pesticides that they have linked to the BEE DEATHS that have been occurring. Our corporate media in America is still doing evening news programs about what in the world is causing the bee deaths? In Europe they have used science, determined the problem, and taken action. Why isn't this happening here? The answer of course is our bought and owned Congress. It is VERY disconcerting that corporations, like Monsanto, control so many members of our Congress, as well as most media. We are in the dark.

NOTES

The Art of Grocery Shopping

Your attitude toward grocery shopping should be positive as well as discriminating. This not a chore, it's a vitally important activity. If you do it properly, it will keep you and your loved ones out of the pharmacy and the doctor's office. We all spend thousands on insurance to protect our homes, cars, and death. To me, grocery shopping is my version of LIFE INSURANCE. If done properly, you will enjoy radiant health and you won't need health insurance to treat chronic illness. Health insurance is supposed to be for accidents, not chronic preventable illness.

Try to start shopping at a local food co-op, if you have one. They are nonprofit food centers that keep more of your money local. This is part of voting with your wallet. Don't give your money to ruthless agribusiness that pollute and give inferior products. I travel thirty-five to forty minutes to my co-op and am GRATEFUL to have one. They are a great resource for locally grown organic food, as well as grass roots efforts to improve the local community. CSA's are also another way to eat organic food. You can sign up for organic foods from local farms. At www.localharvest.org, you can locate what is available in your area. Local farmers markets often have organic produce from local farmers. More conventional grocery stores are carrying organics. The one in my area is not very good, yet. The vegetables and fruit often aren't fresh, because the audience for them is small. I often feel that they put the tired looking organic produce next to the shiny pesticide laden produce so that the comparison is not favorable.

NOTES

However, I buy there when I can, to show there is interest. It must be working because the organic sections are growing.

Even though I live in an apartment, for eight years I have had a container garden. I grow cherry tomatoes, spring mix lettuces, and herbs from May to September. It's fun, easy, saves a little money and tastes AMAZING. I use organic soil and non-gmo seeds that are organic. I do not have a green thumb, but I have had good success with this. If you are luckier than me and have some yard, you can have a real garden. Some of the benefits are: more and better produce, absorbing Vitamin D from being outside, exercise, and fresh air. If you have children, this is a wonderful opportunity to spend quality time and teach them about nutrition, the environment, as well as independence. It's a win-win situation.

Buy as little processed food as you can .The enzymes in LIVE, RAW FOOD are essential to health. Eighty percent of your food should be raw. If you do this, your prep time will be very short. I work every day and cook almost every day. I can prepare dinner in twenty to thirty minutes. It's easy and so delicious. I drink a raw juice at least twice a week. It's the easiest and best way to get a ton of nutrition. Juicing helps control blood sugar, helps to detox your liver and kidneys, delivers beautiful skin, and bright eyes.

I LOVE RAW MILK. I used to think I was lactose intolerant. Apparently, I am only allergic to pasteurized milk. Raw milk is just fine. Apparently, when milk is treated to high temperatures, the proteins are affected and the enzymes are destroyed. I think the body doesn't know what to do with this denatured product. Give it a try and see what you think.

THROW OUT YOUR MICROWAVE! You don't need it. It wrecks the nutrition in your food and exposes you to radiation. Microwaves should never have been permitted for cooking. Microwaves don't save you time, because every minute you think you are saving, will be spent either in a waiting room at the hospital, or, even worse, in a hospital bed. It may be convenient to use a microwave, but it is extremely inconvenient to be sick or have sick kids. This is another lapse

NOTES

by our useless government oversight agencies. REMEMBER, just because it's for sale doesn't mean it's safe or good. In America, you can sell anything, regardless of its harm to us.

Try to introduce some fermented foods into your diet. Live culture yogurts (not the sugary ones, use stevia), live culture sauerkraut and pickles, and assorted vegetables. The word is out that probiotics are necessary for good gut health. This is vital because the majority of our immune cells come from our gut. It is key to a robust immune system. I am going to provide a grid for you to use when grocery shopping for six weeks. Just check off what you are buying for six weeks and try to progressively improve your ratio of raw vs. processed foods. It will make you aware of what you are really buying. If you, or your family, have any health issues, you may be able to resolve them by starting to change what you bring into your house.

BASIC RAW FOODS

Apples	GREEN Lettuce (no iceberg)
Pears	Tomatoes
Raspberries	Broccoli
Strawberries	Green beans
Blackberries	Brussell sprouts
Lemons	Beets
Oranges	Scallions
Pineapple	Onions
Bananas	Carrots
Kiwi	Celery
Plums	Radishes
Pomegranate	Peas
Yams	Parsley
Cucumber	Cabbage
Corn	Bok choy

You can experiment with many other specialty vegetables, especially sea vegetables, which have various health benefits.

NOTES

Raw Nuts
Raw Cheeses:
cheddar, ricotta, cottage
Raw Milk
Raw Yogurt
Organic pastured chicken
Organic olive oil

Grass fed organic beef
Fermented sauerkraut, pickles,
sour crème and yogurt
Organic butter
Organic apple cider vinegar

PROCESSED FOODS

Boxed
cereals
instant dinners
cake and cookies
chips and snacks
frozen dinners
frozen pizza
candy
juice boxes
meat broths
pasta

Canned, Plastic and Jars
vegetables
fruits
jellies and jams
peanut butter
apple sauce
soups and broths
tomato sauce
condiments
soda, juice

Of course this is not a complete list, but you get the idea. Just add on anything not on this list in the category where you think it belongs. Then compute the percentages. The following week try to improve the ratio. For example, if one week you bought cups of applesauce, the following week, BUY THE APPLES. Now, this is where I hear how expensive it is to do this. You must remember, pay less now, and pay thousands later! If you shop well, you will not be at the Pharmacy buying aspirin, Ex-lax, sleep aids, etc. You know why the saying "Eat an apple a day and keep the doctor away" persists? It's because IT'S TRUE! The apple is a little miracle of good news for your body. The white part of the orange is loaded with goodness. When you buy the refined juice, you are losing the majority of the goodness in an orange. Good luck and I hope this will put you on a path of healthy change.

NOTES

GMO Seeds and Food and their Danger to Humanity

Genetically modified organisms are truly the most frightening of the schemes cooked up by corporations to control us. I like to think of Monsanto as the Oil Cartel of food. They want to control the world's food supply as OPEC controls our energy supply, to enrich themselves, and hold all of us hostage. I will try to give you some basic information and show why this corporation should be shut down NOW. I will start with some facts:

1. Monsanto, the creator of Agent Orange, has developed a technology to alter the genetic makeup of seeds. The supposed purpose is to make crops resistant to the effects of herbicides sprayed on plants.
2. Foods produced from GMO seeds now have pesticides INSIDE them. You cannot wash them off.
3. These seeds have not been tested for their effects on humans, as well as animals and the environment. It is an EXPERIMENT.
4. The FDA requires NO INDEPENDENT TESTING of these products.
5. GMO ingredients are now in TWO THIRDS OF OUR FOOD
6. The Supreme Court, FOR THE FIRST TIME, has allowed the patenting of life forms for commercialization.

7. This is an American driven product. Most countries in the rest of the world are greatly alarmed about the use of GMO seed products and foods and have banned them.
8. Independent research is starting to expose the research that the biotech companies have been hiding.
9. Genetic modification actually CUTS the productivity of crops, which contradicts their argument that we need these products to PREVENT food shortages.
10. Independent research shows a direct link between GMO potatoes and cancer in rats. The biotech industry fought eight years in courts, to suppress these studies.
11. GMO corn is shown to cause infertility in mice.
12. Most industrialized nations require GMO labeling of their food. The U.S.A DOES NOT. NINE OF TEN Americans want this labeling. Why don't we have it?
13. Deaths and near deaths have already resulted from GMO foods.
14. Independent research is also showing links between GMO foods and many allergies.
15. GMO crops cause sterility in our soil.
16. Monsanto requires farmers who use their products to pledge not to save seeds, making farmers dependant upon them. Many small farmers in poor countries have committed suicide after their GMO crops have failed, and they weren't permitted any alternative.
17. GMO crops kill beneficial and necessary insects.
18. GMO pollen cannot be contained, and travels the globe via wind, rain, birds, bees, insects, fungus, and bacteria. This genetic pollution cannot be contained.

19. Organic food may not even be possible in the future because of GMO pollution.
20. President Obama has appointed Secretary of Agriculture, Tom Vilsack, a defender of Monsanto.
21. President Obama and his family eat organic food, and are installing an organic garden at the white House. The Bush family also ate organically. This is hypocrisy.
22. The whole point of genetic engineering is to increase sales of chemicals and bio-engineered products to farmers. David Ehrenfield: Professor of Biology, Rutgers University.

Well, isn't this just horrifying? This is a great example of the war I mentioned earlier between us and the corporations. If nine of ten Americans want GMO food labeling, and we don't get it, what does that say about who is really in control of our government? I will be listing the top food distributors in the USA with their phone numbers. Stop buying their stock. Stop buying their products. Make sure to let them know what you are doing and why you are doing it. If we all do it, THEY WILL STOP. We have to make it happen.

NOTES

Genetically Modified Ingredients Overview
As of 07/2007

Currently Commercialized GM Crops in the U.S.:
(Number in parentheses represents the estimated percent that is genetically modified.)

Soy (89%)
Canola (75%)
Hawaiian Papaya (more than 50%)
Tobacco (Quest brand)

Cotton (83%)
Corn (61%)
Alfalfa, zucchini, and yellow squash (small amount)

Other Sources of GMOs:

- Dairy products from cows injected with rbGH
- Food additives, enzymes, flavorings, and processing agents, including the sweetener aspartame (NutraSweet), and rennet used to make hard cheeses
- Meat, eggs, and dairy products from animals that have eaten GM feed
- Honey and bee pollen that may have GM sources of pollen
- Contamination or pollination caused by GM seed or pollen

Some of the Ingredients That May Be Genetically Modified:
Vegetable oil, vegetable fat, and margarines (made with soy, corn, cottonseed, and/or canola).

NOTES

Ingredients derived from soybeans:
Soy flour, soy protein, soy isolates, soy isoflavones, soy lecithin, vegetable proteins, textured vegetable protein (TVP), tofu, tamari, tempeh, and soy protein supplements.

Ingredients derived from corn:
Corn flour, corn gluten, corn masa, corn starch, corn syrup, cornmeal, and High-Fructose Corn Syrup (HFCS).

Some of the Foods That May Contain GM Ingredients:

Infant formula	Salad dressing
Bread	Cereal
Hamburgers and hotdogs	Margarine
Mayonnaise	Crackers
Cookies	Chocolate
Candy	Fried food
Chips	Veggie burgers
Meat substitutes	Ice cream
Frozen Yogurt	Tofu
Tamari	Soy sauce
Tomato sauce	Protein powder
Baking powder (sometimes contains corn starch)	Powdered/Confectioner's sugar (often contains corn starch)
Confectioner's glaze	Alcohol
Vanilla	Powdered sugar
Peanut Butter	Enriched Flour
Vanilla extract (sometimes contains corn syrup)	Pasta
	White vinegar
Malt	

Non-Food Items That May Contain GM Ingredients:

Cosmetics	Soaps
Detergents	Shampoo
Bubble bath	

NOTES

Invisible GM Ingredients

Aspartame	Gluten	Modified Starch
Baking Powder	Glycerides	Monosodium Glutamate (MSG)
Bee Pollen	Glycerin	Oleic Acid
Caramel Color	Glycerol	Phenylalanine
Cellulose	Glycerol monooleate	Phytic acid
Citric acid	Glycine	Sorbitol
Cobalamin (Vitamin B12)	Hemicellulose	Soy flour
Corn gluten	High fructose corn syrup	Soy isolates
Corn masa	Hydrogenated starch	Soy lecithin
Corn oil	Hydrolyzed vegetable protein	Soy protein
Corn syrup	Inositol	Starch
Cornmeal	Incert sugar (colorose or inversol)	Stearic acid
Cornstarch	Tamari	Inverse syrup
Cyclodextrin	Isoflavones	Tempeh
Cystein	Lactic acid	Threonine
Dextrin	Lecithin	Tocopherols (Vitamin E)
Dextrose	Leucine	Tofu
Diacetyl	Lysine	Trehalose
Diglyceride	Malitol	Triglyceride
Fructose	Maltodextrine	Vegetable fat
Fructose (crystalline)	Maltose	Vegetable oil
Glucose	Mannitol	Vitamin B12
Glutamate	Mythlcellulose	Vitamin E
Glutamic acid	Milo starch	Xanthan gum

NOTES

Our understanding is that ascorbic acid (Vitamin C), although usually derived from corn, is probably not GM because it is not made in North America. Honey and bee pollen may contain GMOs if the beehives are near GM crops.

NOTES

Vitamins

Vitamins don't get very much positive press, yet millions, possibly billions of people take them every day. Why is that? I'll give you my take on it. Most people (myself included) take vitamins because they improve our health. We FEEL it. We SEE it. Big Pharma conducts poorly conceived tests that discredit the benefits of specific vitamins, and through the corporate media, gets enormous exposure for the negative research. Vitamins keep us out of hospitals and out of doctor's offices. That is the dilemma of vitamins. They directly impact the profits of the medical establishment. Here's my information list regarding vitamins:

1. Our genes are influenced by our vitamin status. We are not victims of our genes.
2. Doctors (79%) and nurses (89%) use vitamins on a daily basis.
3. Many chronic diseases are caused by specific vitamin deficiencies.
4. Pharmaceutical corporations are purchasing vitamin companies to control the industry. They regularly lobby to make the business climate difficult for vitamin companies.
5. Pharmaceutical drugs are directly responsible for patient deaths. The vitamin industry has an incredible safety record in comparison.
6. Vitamin research conducted by the drug industry invariably use synthetic vitamins with very low dosages.
7. I only use vitamins produced in the USA.

NOTES

8. I only use whole food vitamins.

If you only eat organic food fresh from a nearby source, have very little stress in your life, drink pure clean water and breathe unpolluted air, sleep well every night and regularly exercise, you may not need vitamins. I don't know anybody like that. Vitamins are an essential part of staying well and feeling energetic enough to create a satisfying life. It is my personal belief that the mental and emotional breakdowns we are witnessing in our society are a direct result of vitamin deficiencies. There is a lot of research that demonstrates that many mental problems, like depression and anxiety, disappear when specific nutrients are supplied to the brain.

Each one of us is physically unique. Our mental and spiritual health is not disconnected from our physical health. These aspects of human beings are sophisticated and intertwined. Centuries ago, it was observed that many women after losing a child would contract breast cancer. It was a physical manifestation of heartbreak and grief. Our physical health almost always suffers after an emotional shock. Our common sense tells us this truth. Even ancient peoples observed this. Mental health and physical health will always be connected. It is how we are made. WE ARE NOT MACHINES!

As each of us is unique, our nutritional needs will also vary. Luckily, today, we are able to have our nutritional status analyzed and use the information to right our human ship. I have some guidelines that I have developed through trial and (much) error. I will try to pass on what I have learned to save you money and time.

1. Trust yourself. Only you know how you are feeling. No doctor, expert or other person can tell you how you feel. You are the expert on YOU!
2. Don't take synthetic vitamins. Your body doesn't know what to do with these substances.

NOTES

3. Fillers like magnesium stearates are cheap fillers that actually distract from the absorption and use of the vitamins you need.
4. I recommend only using whole food vitamins. They are like real food and don't require being taken with a meal, so are more useful and more convenient. Megafood and Vitamin Code are two companies that make high quality whole food vitamins.
5. I think everyone would benefit from using Electric Life vitamins for at least THREE months before starting any vitamin regimen. This is an amazing line of nutrients. If I could only afford one of their products, I would use their Factor One. This product efficiently cleanses and tones your digestive tract. It paves the way for the maximum absorption of your food and vitamins. Remember, it is what you absorb that counts
6. It helps a lot to find a good homeopath to work with you while you work through your health issues. Homeopathy is the system of medicine used by the Queen of England. It doesn't get much respect here in the states because of the control of the media by Big Pharma. I can testify as to its usefulness. IT WORKS. IT'S INEXPENSIVE. IT'S SAFE. I can see why the Queen uses it. A truly skilled homeopath will use a mixture of homeopathic tinctures, herbs and vitamins to treat you. If they don't use herbs and vitamins, look for someone else. Regardless of what ANY health professional advises me, I do my own homework. With the internet you can look up anything and find out the lowdown on any product that is recommended. Read the risks, be informed and take control of your health.

NOTES

7. I take periodic breaks from my supplements. This way I can evaluate if they are working. Usually after taking a certain supplement for three or four months, I will pause for three weeks and see how I feel. If I start to feel tired, have trouble sleeping or any other feeling crops up, I know that the vitamins were helping and I resume them. I switch brands every twelve months or so, to prevent any allergies. Many herbs should be used two or three weeks at a time with a two month break. Herbal effects will peter out if taken too long.

NOTES

Air

Of all the aspects of improving your health, this one is more challenging because we are at the mercy of our own industrial society. Despite this dreary scenario, there ARE things you can do to protect yourself and your family. As you may have heard, the air in your home is so important because so much time is spent at home. I have placed air filters where I spend the most time, such as the living/family room and the bedroom. There are many types of filters out there with various price points. I will list some sources in Air Solutions. If you work outside the home, think about the risks there. Think about the equipment that surrounds you. Is any of it hazardous to your lungs? Are you in your car, a plane, or truck a big portion of your day? There are solutions for these places, if they are a large portion of your day.

There is general air pollution that is outside your control, and then there is air pollution that you DO control. I'm talking about the items you buy, that off gas into the air of your home. Cleaning products, air fresheners, paint, toxic furnishings and personal care products absorbed through the skin are just some of the hazards. This is a part of your "democracy spending". You can "vote" for products that are safe. As I said at the beginning of this book, it took me two years to clear out the old toxic products and replace them with new healthy products. Even with supposedly "green" products, there is a lot of scamming going on. I will offer sources for products I have tried that are superior to conventional toxic products, and work even better. I'm pretty tough regarding chemicals. I am a purist, as I don't tolerate anything resembling an artificial chemical in what I use to keep my house and body clean. I set a high bar because I feel it is VITAL to my well being to be careful and I don't want to deal with this crap, so I don't want it around! The added benefit to this change is that most of the companies I buy from are American companies. I want to "vote" for American workers and small entrepreneurs when I lay down my hard earned money!

Many of my prior suggestions regarding water and food also relate to the issue of air pollution. When you clean your shower water and eat nutritious food, you are relieving the toxic burden of your body. This means that your lungs can detox the bad air you encounter more easily because the total toxic burden is smaller.

Air Solutions

1. Buy some indoor plants. NASA did a study to find out which plants were best to filter air at the space station. The following list of plants absorbs carbon dioxide, and creates oxygen, as well as removing dangerous chemicals in your home. Check online, or with a local nursery, to determine which plants will work best in your local climate and environment.

THE LIST

- English Ivy
- Spider Plant
- Golden Pothos
- Peace Lily
- Chinese Evergreen
- Bamboo Palm
- Snake Plant
- Heartleaf Philodendron
- Selloum Philodendron
- Elephant Ear Philodendron
- Red-edged Dracaena
- Cornstalk Dracaena
- Janet Craig Dracaena
- Warneck Dracaena
- Weeping Fig
- Gerbera Daisy
- Pot Mum
- Rubber Plant

NOTES

Also check for any toxicity if you have small children or pets, before you purchase any plant.

2. Buy an air filter. There are a variety of air filters available. The first one you buy should be placed where you spend the most time. Buy additional filters for other rooms as you can afford them.
3. Some resources for this topic are the book HOW TO GROW FRESH AIR by www.equinoxproducts.com

How to Survive (and Thrive) in a Toxic World

NOTES

Parents of Infants and Young Children

Body Burden — The Pollution in Newborns

A benchmark investigation of industrial chemicals, pollutants and pesticides in umbilical cord blood

Environmental Working Group, July 14, 2005

Summary. In the month leading up to a baby's birth, the umbilical cord pulses with the equivalent of at least 300 quarts of blood each day, pumped back and forth from the nutrient- and oxygen-rich placenta to the rapidly growing child cradled in a sac of amniotic fluid. This cord is a lifeline between mother and baby, bearing nutrients that sustain life and propel growth.

Not long ago scientists thought that the placenta shielded cord blood — and the developing baby — from most chemicals and pollutants in the environment. But now we know that at this critical time when organs, vessels, membranes and systems are knit together from single cells to finished form in a span of weeks, the umbilical cord carries not only the building blocks of life, but also a steady stream of industrial chemicals, pollutants and pesticides that cross the placenta as readily as residues from cigarettes and alcohol. This is the human "body burden" — the pollution in people that permeates everyone in the world, including babies in the womb.

In a study spearheaded by the Environmental Working Group (EWG) in collaboration with Commonweal, researchers at two major laboratories found an average of 200 industrial chemicals and pollutants in umbilical cord blood from 10 babies born in August and September of 2004 in U.S. hospitals. Tests revealed a total of 287 chemicals in the group. The umbilical cord blood of these 10 children, collected by Red Cross after the cord was cut, harbored pesticides, consumer product ingredients, and wastes from burning coal, gasoline, and garbage.

This study represents the first reported cord blood tests for 261 of the targeted chemicals and the first reported detections in cord blood for 209 compounds. Among them are eight perfluorochemicals used as stain and oil repellants in fast food packaging, clothes and textiles — including the Teflon chemical PFOA, recently characterized as a likely human carcinogen by the EPA's Science Advisory Board — dozens of widely used brominated flame retardants and their toxic by-products; and numerous pesticides.

Of the 287 chemicals we detected in umbilical cord blood, we know that 180 cause cancer in humans or animals, 217 are toxic to the brain and nervous system, and 208 cause birth defects or abnormal development in animal tests. The dangers of pre- or post-natal exposure to this complex mixture of carcinogens, developmental toxins and neurotoxins have never been studied.

Chemicals and pollutants detected in human umbilical cord blood

Hg

Mercury (Hg) - tested for 1, found 1

Pollutant from coal-fired power plants, mercury-containing products, and certain industrial processes. Accumulates in seafood. Harms brain development and function.

PAH

Polyaromatic hydrocarbons (PAHs) - tested for 18, found 9

Pollutants from burning gasoline and garbage. Linked to cancer. Accumulates in food chain.

BD/F

Polybrominated dibenzodioxins and furans (PBDD/F) - tested for 12, found 7

Contaminants in brominated flame retardants. Pollutants and byproducts from plastic production and incineration. Accumulate in food chain. Toxic to developing endocrine (hormone) system

PFC

Perfluorinated chemicals (PFCs) - tested for 12, found 9

Active ingredients or breakdown products of Teflon, Scotchgard, fabric and carpet protectors, food wrap coatings. Global contaminants. Accumulate in the environment and the food chain. Linked to cancer, birth defects, and more.

D/F

Polychlorinated dibenzodioxins and furans (PCDD/F) - tested for 17, found 11

Pollutants, by-products of PVC production, industrial bleaching, and incineration. Cause cancer in humans. Persist for decades in the environment. Very toxic to developing endocrine (hormone) system.

OC

Organochlorine pesticides (OCs) - tested for 28, found 21

DDT, chlordane and other pesticides. Largely banned in the

U.S. Persist for decades in the environment. Accumulate up the food chain, to man. Cause cancer and numerous reproductive effects.

Polybrominated diphenyl ethers (PBDEs) - tested for 46, found 32

Flame retardant in furniture foam, computers, and televisions. Accumulates in the food chain and human tissues. Adversely affects brain development and the thyroid.

Polychlorinated Naphthalenes (PCNs) - tested for 70, found 50

Wood preservatives, varnishes, machine lubricating oils, waste incineration. Common PCB contaminant. Contaminate the food chain. Cause liver and kidney damage.

Polychlorinated biphenyls (PCBs) - tested for 209, found 147

Industrial insulators and lubricants. Banned in the U.S. in 1976. Persist for decades in the environment. Accumulate up the food chain, to man. Cause cancer and nervous system problems.

Source: Chemical analyses of 10 umbilical cord blood samples were conducted by AXYS Analytical Services (Sydney, BC) and Flett Research Ltd. (Winnipeg, MB).

Chemical exposures in the womb or during infancy can be dramatically more harmful than exposures later in life. Substantial scientific evidence demonstrates that children face amplified risks from their body burden of pollution; the findings are particularly strong for many of the chemicals found in this study, including mercury, PCBs and dioxins. Children's vulnerability derives from both rapid development and incomplete defense systems:

- A developing child's chemical exposures are greater pound-for-pound than those of adults.

- An immature, porous blood-brain barrier allows greater chemical exposures to the developing brain.
- Children have lower levels of some chemical-binding proteins, allowing more of a chemical to reach "target organs."
- A baby's organs and systems are rapidly developing, and thus are often more vulnerable to damage from chemical exposure.
- Systems that detoxify and excrete industrial chemicals are not fully developed.
- The longer future life span of a child compared to an adult allows more time for adverse effects to arise.

The 10 children in this study were chosen randomly, from among 2004's summer season of live births from mothers in Red Cross' volunteer, national cord blood collection program. They were not chosen because their parents work in the chemical industry or because they were known to bear problems from chemical exposures in the womb. Nevertheless, each baby was born polluted with a broad array of contaminants.

U.S. industries manufacture and import approximately 75,000 chemicals, 3,000 of them at over a million pounds per year. Health officials do not know how many of these chemicals pollute fetal blood and what the health consequences of *in utero* exposures may be.

Had we tested for a broader array of chemicals, we would almost certainly have detected far more than 287. But testing umbilical cord blood for industrial chemicals is technically challenging. Chemical manufacturers are not required to divulge to the public or government health officials methods to detect their chemicals in humans. Few labs are equipped with the machines and expertise to run the tests or the funding to develop the methods. Laboratories have yet to develop methods to test human tissues for the vast majority of chemicals on the market, and the few tests that labs are able to conduct are expensive. Laboratory costs for the cord blood analyses reported here were $10,000 per sample.

A developing baby depends on adults for protection, nutrition, and, ultimately, survival. As a society we have a responsibility to ensure that babies do not enter this world pre-polluted, with 200 industrial chemicals in their blood. Decades-old bans on a handful of chemicals like PCBs, lead gas additives, DDT and other pesticides have led to significant declines in people's blood levels of these pollutants. But good news like this is hard to find for other chemicals.

The Toxic Substances Control Act, the 1976 federal law meant to ensure the safety of commercial chemicals, essentially deemed 63,000 existing chemicals "safe as used" the day the law was passed, through mandated, *en masse* approval for use with no safety scrutiny. It forces the government to approve new chemicals within 90 days of a company's application at an average pace of seven per day. It has not been improved for nearly 30 years — longer than any other major environmental or public health statute — and does nothing to reduce or ensure the safety of exposure to pollution in the womb.

Because the Toxic Substances Control Act fails to mandate safety studies, the government has initiated a number of voluntary programs to gather more information about chemicals, most notably the high production volume (HPV) chemical screening program. But these efforts have been largely ineffective at reducing human exposures to chemicals. They are no substitute for a clear statutory requirement to protect children from the toxic effects of chemical exposure.

In light of the findings in this study and a substantial body of supporting science on the toxicity of early life exposures to industrial chemicals, we strongly urge that federal laws and policies be reformed to ensure that children are protected from chemicals, and that to the maximum extent possible, exposures to industrial chemicals before birth be eliminated. The sooner society takes action, the sooner we can reduce or end pollution in the womb.

Tests show 287 industrial chemicals in 10 newborn babies

Pollutants include consumer product ingredients, banned industrial chemicals and pesticides, and waste byproducts

Sources and uses of chemicals in newborn blood	Chemical family name	Total number of chemicals found in 10 newborns (range in individual babies)
Common consumer product chemicals (and their breakdown products)		**47 chemicals** (23 - 38)
Pesticides, actively used in U.S.	Organochlorine pesticides (OCs)	7 chemicals (2 - 6)
Stain and grease resistant coatings for food wrap, carpet, furniture (Teflon, Scotchgard, Stainmaster...)	Perfluorochemicals (PFCs)	8 chemicals (4 - 8)
Fire retardants in TVs, computers, furniture	Polybrominated diphenyl ethers (PBDEs)	32 chemicals (13 - 29)
Chemicals banned or severely restricted in the U.S. (and their breakdown products)		**212 chemicals** (111 - 185)
Pesticides, phased out of use in U.S.	Organochlorine pesticides (OCs)	14 chemicals (7 - 14)

Stain and grease resistant coatings for food wrap, carpet, furniture (pre-2000 Scotchgard)	Perfluorochemicals (PFCs)	1 chemicals (1 - 1)
Electrical insulators	Polychlorinated biphenyls (PCBs)	147 chemicals (65 - 134)
Broad use industrial chemicals - flame retardants, pesticides, electrical insultators	Polychlorinated naphthalenes (PCNs)	50 chemicals (22 - 40)
Waste byproducts		**28 chemicals (6 - 21)**
Garbage incineration and plastic production wastes	Polychlorinated and Polybrominated dibenzo dioxins and furans (PCDD/F and PBDD/F)	18 chemicals (5 - 13)
Car emissions and other fossil fuel combustion	Polynuclear aromatic hydrocarbons (PAHs)	10 chemicals (1 - 10)
Power plants (coal burning)	Methylmercury	1 chemicals (1 - 1)
All chemicals found		**287 chemicals (154 - 231)**

Source: Environmental Working Group analysis of tests of 10 umbilical cord blood samples conducted by AXYS Analytical Services (Sydney, BC) and Flett Research Ltd. (Winnipeg, MB).

Parents of Infants and Young Children

    I wanted to have a short chapter directed to parents, and potential parents, of our youngest and most vulnerable population. I cringe now at the information provided (and NOT provided) by my obstetrician and pediatrician. When I was pregnant with my daughter, they had misinformed me about so many things regarding keeping Brett healthy. I don't think they were malicious, just ignorant. They just passed on what they had learned in medical school, and so much of it is WRONG! Again, I'll do one of the little lists you have been reading throughout this book:

1. Breast feeding is incredibly SUPERIOR to any other food for newborns. Nothing else even comes close. I will always regret not breastfeeding Brett. My pediatrician said it didn't matter, and I stupidly believed her.
2. Any vaccines given at birth are OBSCENE, and should be considered CRIMINAL with appropriate punishment. Some states are mandating the Hepatitis B vaccine at birth. This is nothing but a blatant money grab by pharmaceutical corporations. This vaccine supposedly protects a child from a sexually transmitted disease for SEVEN YEARS. I guess the promiscuous infant situation needed attention!
3. Today, babies are being born with a toxic chemical load. The potential harm from a vaccine injection of chemicals, and God knows what else, is highly irresponsible. They are injected without the GOOD REASONING that should be carefully considered by parents.
4. The research is showing increasing damage from vaccines. For instance, Hepatitis B is linked to male development disability. There are THOUSANDS of studies showing various problems caused by vaccines. Many of them

aren't done in the USA because of the unprecedented power of Pharmaceutical Corporations. American research is really a great example of the fox running the hen house. They pay for research that is biased and useless to promote their damaging products for money.
5. The CDC has FINALLY put out a statement that mothers should not use tap water to mix infant formula, because it harms a child's I.Q. I guess it is just dandy for children's brains after formula is stopped. It is no accident that nature does not include fluoride in breast milk. Is the ADD problem really a fluoride problem?
6. Children's bodies are much more susceptible to toxins than are adult bodies. It is important to use organic products for children including baby powder, shampoos, etc. Plastic and babies don't mix!

Your child depends on you to do the right thing and protect them from the corporations who want to exploit their needs for money. YOU are their firewall. Don't protect your computer better than you protect your baby. They are helpless. I had a very hard time with myself after Brett got so seriously sick. Unknowingly, I helped make her sick because I listened to the "experts" instead of looking into things for my self.

Buddha said it best: "Do not believe in anything simply because you have heard it. Do not believe in anything because it is spoken and rumored by many. Do not believe in anything because it is written in your religious books. Do not believe in anything merely on the authority of your teachers and elders. Do not believe in traditions because they have been handed down for many generations. Only after your own observation and analysis, when you find that anything agrees with reason and is conducive to the benefit of one and all, then accept it and live up to it".

To exemplify this quote is the history of hand washing prior to medical treatment. Today it is a given that medical staff should wash their hands before interacting with patients. However, this was not always so. Dr. Ignaz Semmelweis of Hungary, in the early 1850's, wrote a book about his observation that washing one's hands prior to childbirth greatly decreased the death and illness rates among mothers and newborns. His work was greeted with scorn from the "experts" of the day. He was so greatly harassed that he had a nervous breakdown and died in an insane asylum.

I believe that in the future, people will look with horror upon the vaccines we forced on children, as well as the deadly chemicals injected into the veins of cancer patients. We are still, today, in the Dark Ages of medicine, despite advances in trauma care. Treatment of chronic diseases is ineffective, and regarding cancer, it is brutal.

Vaccines

I know there is a lot of angst going on in the world regarding vaccine safety. The reason I am getting into the fray is that as I researched treatments and information to help my daughter, it became clear that neither the government nor Big Pharma have been truthful about vaccine damage. They present vaccines as miracle drugs with almost no down side. I was shocked that doctors ARE NOT REQUIRED TO REPORT vaccine damage. This has led to almost no good information regarding the harm caused by vaccines. I discovered that the polio vaccine may have played a role in the type of cancer Brett contracted. I will try to keep this story short, even though there is a lot to know. Entire books have been written about it.

Back in the early sixties, like millions of children (ninety-eight million to be exact), I received the polio vaccine. Unknown to all of us, was the fact that these doses were contaminated with a green monkey virus called Simian Virus 40, or SV40. The degree of contamination varied. As a resident of Pittsburgh, PA, I received some of the most contaminated doses. This is an example of a lie knowingly told to us by the government as well as Big Pharma. Even today, despite news to the contrary, this is still the line they use. Vaccines are safe. Problems are rare. Actually, the government and pharmaceutical corporations have never conducted any study into the after effects of SV40 contamination, SO WE DON'T KNOW. It is an impossible statement that they have uttered. First, I will give you a little information about SV40. It is used in cancer research because it is considered "A LITTLE CANCER WAR MACHINE". It

NOTES

produces tumors in animals faster than any other virus used in research. I was shocked that this type of virus was not considered worthy of study to determine its harm to the millions of children who received it. There should have been long term studies done to know what the consequences were, and are, regarding this vaccine.

The most recent developments that have turned up are disturbing. It turns out that this virus is turning up in rare childhood cancers. Yes, they are finding this virus in bone tumors like my daughters. The scary thing is that BRETT NEVER RECEIVED THE POLIO VACCINE. Apparently, it is possible that these children with osteosarcoma had to have inherited the virus. As cancer incidence is exploding among people under 40, is this the reason? The incidence of bone tumors in children has increased FORTY PER CENT IN TEN YEARS. Again, my common sense tells me that the safety of vaccines is far from a sure thing. Why would the government perpetuate the lie? Until the government comes clean, I would not trust their vaccine assurances. They don't deserve our trust. This virus is also turning up in mesothelioma. Like me, I am sure you have seen the television commercials by lawyers for mesothelioma law suits. Is there another aspect to this disease besides asbestos?

Brett also received the Hepatitis B vaccine six months prior to her osteosarcoma diagnosis. Her surgeon told me that the tumor started six months before her diagnosis. Like many parents, our common sense tells us that there is some type of relationship between getting a vaccine and the start of disease. Just because the medical community doesn't understand the relationship, does not mean that it doesn't exist. Prior to that Hepatitis series of shots, she was normal and vigorous, and then six months later she was in a fight for her life.

This vaccination decision is still yours, except in New Jersey & Maryland, where parents have lost their say. This is an ominous sign. The state deciding the treatments our children receive gives me a chill up the spine. I think it's

NOTES

disgusting and immoral. Some simple facts regarding vaccination: There are populations that don't vaccinate, and their children are FINE. It is impossible to vaccinate against every pathogen that exists. That's why God gave us an immune system. On a daily basis, our immune system disposes of thousands of pathogens and we aren't even aware of it. If you follow my lead regarding the recommendations in this book, you will have a robust immune system that can handle almost anything, except perhaps the deadly pathogens that our government likes to dream up, at our expense!

I have included a copy of a form that you can present to your pediatrician. As you know, when we seek treatment we have to sign away our rights. I don't think it is out of line to demand the same from those who provide us health services. If nothing else, you may have a lively discussion of these issues and learn what type of person to whom you are entrusting your child's life.

HERE'S THE FORM:

NOTES

Vaccine Warranty Form

Please ask your doctor to sign this if he/she thinks Vaccines are safe.

Physician's Warranty of Vaccine Safety

I (physician's name, degree), _____
am a physician licensed to practice medicine in the State of_____, and my DEA number is _____.
My medical specialty is _____.

I have a thorough understanding of the risks and benefits of all the medications that I prescribe for, or administer, to my patients.
In the case of (Patient's name) _____, age __, whom I have examined, I find that certain risk factors exist that I justify the recommended vaccinations.

The following is a list of said risk factors and the vaccinations that will protect against them:
Risk Factor Vaccination:

_____
_____
_____
_____

_____

I am aware that vaccines typically contain many of the following fillers:

- aluminum hydroxide
- aluminum phosphate
- ammonium sulfate
- amphotericin B
- animal tissues : pig blood, horse blood, rabbit brain, dog kidney, monkey kidney, chick embryo, chicken egg, duck egg
- calf (bovine) serum
- betapropiolactone
- fetal bovine serum
- formaldehyde
- formalin
- gelatin
- glycerol
- human diploid cells (originating from human aborted fetal tissue)
- hydrolyzed gelatin
- mercury thimerosol
- monosodium glutamate (MSG)
- neomycin
- neomycin sulfate
- phenol red indicator
- phenoxyethanol (antifreeze)
- potassium diphosphate
- potassium monophosphate
- polymyxin B
- polysorbate 20
- polysorbate 80
- porcine (pig) pancreatic hydrolysate of casein
- residual MRC5 proteins
- sorbitol
- sucrose
- tri(n)butylphosphate, VERO cells, a continuous line of monkey kidney cells, and washed sheep red blood

and, hereby, warrant that these ingredients are safe for injection into the body of my patient. Reports to the contrary, such as reports that mercury thimerosol causes severe neurological and immunological damage, are not credible. I am aware that some vaccines have been found to have been contaminated with Simian Virus 40 (SV-40) and that SV-40 is casually linked by some researchers to non-Hodgkin's lymphoma and mesotheliomas in humans as well as in experimental animals.

I hereby give my assurance that the vaccines I employ in my practice do not contain SV-40 or any other live viruses. (Alternately, I hereby give my assurance that said SV-40 or other viruses pose no substantive risk to my patient). I hereby warrant that the vaccines I am recommending for the care of (Patient's name)
Do not contain any cells from aborted human babies (also known as "fetuses").

In order to protect my patient's well being, I have taken the following steps to guarantee that the vaccines I will use will contain no damaging contaminants.
Steps taken:

_____
_____
_____
_____
_____

I have personally investigated the reports made to the VAERS (Vaccine Adverse Event Reporting System) and state that it is my professional opinion that the vaccines I am recommending are safe for administration to a child under the age of 5 years.
The bases for my opinion are itemized on Exhibit A, attached hereto, "Physician's Bases for Professional Opinion of Vaccine Safety." (Please itemize each recommended vaccine separately

along with the bases for arriving at the conclusion that the vaccine is safe for administration to a child under the age of 5 years.)
The professional journal articles I have relied upon in the issuance of this Physician's Warranty of Vaccine Safety are itemized on Exhibit B, attached hereto, "Scientific Articles in Support of Physician's Warranty of Vaccine Safety". The professional journal articles that I have read which contain opinions adverse to my opinion are itemized on Exhibit C, attached hereto, "Scientific Articles Contrary to Physician's Opinion of vaccine Safety." The reasons for my determining that thee articles in Exhibit C were invalid are delineated in Attachment D, attached hereto, "Physician's Reasons for Determining the Invalidity of Adverse Scientific Opinions."

Hepatitis B:
I understand that 60% of patients who are vaccinated for Hepatitis B will lose detectable antibodies to Hepatitis B within 12 years. I understand that in 1996, only 54 cases of Hepatitis B were reported to the CDC on the 0-1 year age group. I understand that in the VAERS, there were 1,080 total reports of adverse reactions from Hepatitis B vaccine in 1996 in the 0-1 age group, with 47 deaths reported. I understand that 50% of patients who contract Hepatitis B develop no symptoms after exposure, I understand that 30% will develop only flu-like symptoms and will have lifetime immunity.

I understand that 20% will develop the symptoms of the disease, but that 95% will fully recover and have lifetime immunity. I understand that 5% of the patients who are exposed to Hepatitis B will become chronic carriers of the disease. I understand that 75% of the chronic carriers will live with an asymptomatic infection and that 25% of the chronic carriers will develop chronic liver disease or liver cancer, 10-30 years after the acute infection. The following studies have been performed to demonstrate the safety of the Hepatitis B vaccine in children under the age of 5 years:

Vaccine Warranty Form

In addition to the recommended vaccinations as protections against the above cited risk factors, I have recommended other non-vaccine measures to protect the health of my patient and have enumerated said non-vaccine measures on Exhibit D, attached hereto, "Non-Vaccine Measures to Protect Against Risk Factors."

I am issuing this Physician's Warranty of Vaccine Safety in my professional capacity as the attending physician to (Patient's Name) _____.
Regardless of the legal entity under which I normally practice medicine, I am issuing this statement in both my business and individual capacities and hereby waive any statutory, Common Law, Constitutional, UCC, International Treaty, and any other legal immunities from liable lawsuits in the instant case. I issue this document of my own free will after consultation with competent legal counsel, whose name is _____, An attorney admitted to the Bar in the State of _____.

_____(Name of Attending (Physician)
_____L.S.

_____(Signature of Attending Physician)

Signed on this _____ day of _____ _____A.D.

Witness:_____ Date:_____

Notary Public:_____ Date:_____

NOTES

How Cancer Cures are Suppressed or Ignored by Pharmaceutical Corporations, Universities, Doctors, and Researchers

One of the most devastating moments (there were so many) during the last eight years was when I discovered that Brett's disease, osteosarcoma, was cured over thirty years ago. It is a crushing blow to realize that Brett, and our family, could have been spared the horror of current cancer treatment for osteosarcoma. I have tried, very diligently, to expose the truth about this cure for osteosarcoma, with almost no cooperation from the legal profession or the media. Here is the story that they have refused to print or litigate.

In the early seventies, a teenager, Linda LeCam, was diagnosed with osteosarcoma in her leg. Her father was a very famous mathematician at Berkeley, in California. His name was Lucien LeCam. Upon receiving this devastating diagnosis, he immediately put his skills to work to try and save his daughter's life. Amazingly, HE DID! That's just GREAT, isn't it? Yes, it was great for Linda and the other sixteen participants, but what about the thousands of other children who did not have the access that she and her family had to deal with this terrible problem? For the rest of us it has not been great. In fact, it is a mountain of tragedy for the rest of us.

As I had investigated Linda's story, it became apparent that something was very wrong. There is no media article that I can find declaring the amazing news that children were cured of this STILL incurable disease. The fact is that LINDA SHOULD NOT STILL BE WITH US, BUT SHE IS! Don't get me wrong, I am thrilled that Linda is alive and enjoying her life today, I just don't understand why no one else was afforded the same gift. Linda underwent typical treatment for osteosarcoma. Her diseased leg was amputated. She also had tumors in her lungs and had lung surgery to remove them. This also is typical for this osteosarcoma. The prognosis for a child who continues to get tumors in the lungs is STILL very poor. I imagine it was even more dire back in the early seventies. Yet, she is still with us!

Linda was added to a clinical trial for children with osteosarcoma at Berkeley, where her father was a professor. The clinical trial was designed to use immunotherapy (vaccine therapy) to try to control the disease. Many people don't realize that vaccine therapy for cancer has been around for a LOOOOOOONG time. Today, we see television commercials for cancer vaccines and they are presented as something NEW in the war against cancer, BUT THEY ARE NOT NEW. The vaccine, developed for Linda and the other sixteen children enrolled, involved the use of TRANSFER FACTOR. This is a substance, also found in breast milk for infants, that confers immunity from mother to child. There were five physicians involved in this clinical trial. I communicated with one, Dr. Vera Byers. I could not locate the other three and the fifth doctor had been MURDERED. By the time I am through telling you this true story, you will feel as if you are watching a Lifetime movie. It's so surreal because it really happened. Dr. Vera Byers was not particularly helpful. Like most doctors, I found her cold and not very empathetic. My daughter's life was on the line, yet her reluctance to help was palpable. In our first conversation I brought up Linda's ordeal. Right away her tone changed and it became clear that this was very personal to her. She said Linda was SO VERY SICK. Linda wasn't just very sick. Linda WAS DYING. So how did they save Linda and the other children? This is where it gets sticky. She didn't want to talk about it. I had also contacted Linda by email, as she is now also a professor, like her father, I explained to her that Brett was suffering from the same disease and we needed to know what she had done to be brought back from death. She also did not want to discuss it. Is it just me or is this not the strangest of situations? Today, when someone is brought back from the jaws of death, IT'S BIG NEWS. I felt that what was accomplished in this clinical trial was VERY BIG NEWS! Seventeen children cured of deadly cancer using vaccine therapy. Even today that would be a shot heard round the world. WHY WASN'T IT? Sadly, I suspect it was that $25,000 a week we were paying for Brett's treatment. Cancer treatment is the sacred cow of modern medicine. The money, jobs, and economies dependent upon this disease WERE enormous, and ARE enormous. No little vaccine was going to get in the way of this cash cow.

    I was forced to hire a few detectives to get more information about this situation, as Dr. Byers and Linda LeCam refused to give any more responses to the many questions I had. I found out who funded the clinical trial and also more information about the murdered doctor. The other three doctors I could not find. I tried to find an attorney to tackle this case. I strongly feel that if a cure for cancer was discovered and then suppressed for money, which should be brought out into the light. The devastation caused by the suppression of this vital information is truly staggering. Millions of people die everyday from cancer. There are very few families untouched by cancer. Trillions of dollars have been spent without very much success. It could transform the world to finally offer a solution to this devastating disease.

Sadly, I believe the cure fir cancer will come from courtrooms, and not research labs. What a testament to how screwed up corporations and governments have become.

The Rewards of Change

Like most humans, I HATE CHANGE! I enjoy being in my comfort zone. Change, even good change, always instills a little fear. We hug the familiar to our chests, just like the little blankies many of us dragged around the house as small children. However, this book is directed to adults, who are now responsible for themselves, and may be responsible for their children as well. I am hoping that you can see, after reading what I have to say, that your fear of the ill health you may suffer, will overcome your innate fear of change. I want to put you in the driver's seat. I don't want you to be blindsided. I don't want you and your family to suffer as we have suffered.

When you undertake my suggestions, you will be in control of your health. Hospitals, doctors and pharmacies won't take over your life. Financially, you will not be victimized. As the fluoride haze dissipates from your mind, you will feel the sense of freedom and control that you had as a young person. A great burden will have been lifted, a burden of which you may not even have been aware. You won't be tired. You will be more creative with clear thinking. If you have children, you will experience the joy of their health and vitality. I can hardly describe the exquisite pain of watching a beloved child suffer. There are no words. I couldn't wish it upon anyone. You will rediscover your love of food as you transition to organics, because organic food is DELICIOUS and SATISFYING, as it is not void of nutrients. You will save money because you will not purchase or tolerate the toxic products on the market. As more people refuse inferior food and harmful products, corporations will change their ways and produce products that enhance humanity, not harm it. In your own way, by the small decisions you make every day, you are helping to create a better world for yourself as well as future generations, and that is as it should be. GOOD LUCK!

Citizen Responsibility

As you finish this book, you can see I do quite a bit of finger pointing. However, the biggest finger is pointed at me. All of this greed and subterfuge carried on by ruthless corporations and the government they control happens because of citizen neglect, lack of attention, and opposition from me and millions of voting Americans. Our hands off approach, and disinterest regarding the running of America, have allowed the deterioration of our society to occur.

One thing I discovered, as I moved back toward true health, is a strength and energy to actively participate in this Democratic Experiment called the United States of America. I didn't have the will, or health, to get involved in these vital issues before I changed my life. Maybe the plan of corporations like Monsanto, and the government they control, is to slowly cripple us so we do not have the energy to object to their nefarious practices. It certainly appears to be so. I hope you will find, after a year or so, when you are feeling better, that you will start to act and get involved in running this country and pushing back. It is more than time to show these uncaring corporations that the party is over, and we refuse to live in the world they want to control. It isn't difficult to do. First, vote with your wallet. I regularly contact my representatives in Congress about the issues I care about. These phone calls DO matter. Participate in groups who have your viewpoint. Let corporations know what you think of their practices. When you reject a product they make, LET THEM KNOW. The organic food section at my local market has quadrupled in the last year. Money is their God, and they will respond accordingly. Let your friends and family know what you are doing. Be the change you want to see. I firmly believe that each of us has a God given genius that can fix any problem and create a magnificent world.

Toxins of the Mind and Spirit

Just in case you haven't caught on, it is increasingly obvious that our government and the corporations that control it, constantly work together to keep the average American FAT, STUPID, SICKLY and POOR. I have discussed in previous chapters how they are doing this, and in this chapter I want to discuss your state of mind and how important it is to protect and nourish it. There is a definite connection between the mind (or soul) and our physical health. I feel they are symbiotic aspects of the total picture of human health.

Just as toxic pharmaceutical drugs and poor nutrition affect the functioning of the brain and our behavior, toxic thoughts also can manifest physical symptoms. Sadness and depression suppress our immune systems. Constant negative influences impact our state of mind.

Here are a few questions and observations. Our corporate driven media is mostly focused on the negative behavior of people. If an alien landed on earth and was only allowed to watch and listen to mainstream media and not interact with us, they would think we were all murderers, rapists, thieves, sexual deviants with little intelligence, and riddled with FEAR. The truth is that the majority of people are responsible, hardworking, kind, patriotic people who believe in a Creator by some name.

MOST PEOPLE ARE GOOD.

Why do the media want to portray us as opposite to what most of us are? What purpose does it serve to have people think in a negative way about themselves and others? I think it is to profit and maintain control over us. I look around the world and I don't like what I see. I want to live in a world where I don't have to lock up my house and my car, where I don't have to fear my neighbor. I want a world free of nuclear dangers and instant annihilation. I want to live free to pursue my dreams and help create the paradise that God intended for ALL of us. I am not a fool or a Pollyanna. We don't have the world which is our true destiny because people have given up on this idea as a goal.

Start today and work to insulate yourself and your family from these heavily harmful trends in media. Fill your mind with uplifting material and you will not allow depression to paralyze your good intentions and handicap your health. I believe this is a Universe created for and by love. I think you will find that the more you give out to others, the more you help yourself. This philosophy has multiplied positive action and in return the Universe fulfills our dearest wishes in astonishing ways.

This is a world that humans have created, not some sort of Satan or Devil. This world is a reflection of our own thoughts and actions. If we don't like what we see, we should change our thoughts. When our thinking changes, our actions will change and the world will change. For thousands of years, the human race has been governed by fear. I think it is past time to grow up, stop being fearful, and fulfill our destiny. We have the power to create a beautiful new world, one thought and one action at a time. Exciting, isn't it?

Brett's Story

(Warning: Very Troubling, and Emotional Aspects)

Early in March 2001, my thirteen year old daughter, Brett, came home limping after track practice complaining of pain in her right knee. The next day I drove her to school and watched her limp her way to the building entrance. A terrible sense of foreboding came over me. I believe maternal instincts are infallible, so I scheduled an appointment with an orthopedic specialist the next day. He x-rayed her leg and there was a 2cm. tumor growing at the end of Brett's right femur, osteosarcoma's most favored site. With this extremely distressing news, we had just received first class tickets to the World of Childhood Cancer.

Imagine that your pediatrician states "your daughter now has ADD and she won't be getting A's in school anymore, she will be lucky to get C's." How would a parent feel? Or perhaps the doctor says "your son is partially deaf," "Your daughter's heart is damaged" "Your son's liver is damaged;" "Your daughter's leg needs to be amputated," "Your son's arm needs to be amputated." Hearing any ONE of these statements would create trauma for a parent. Being told ALL AT ONCE is a catastrophe of unbelievable proportions. Welcome to the world of osteosarcoma and chemotherapy. The pharmaceutical companies brag about the success of chemotherapy in dealing with childhood cancer. These side effects are what they are proud of, what they proclaim as success.

Osteosarcoma is a tough disease which, in America, gets very brutal treatment. I denote 'IN AMERICA' BECAUSE THIS IS THE WORST PLACE TO BE IF THE DIAGNOSIS IS THIS TYPE OF CANCER. In America, a cancer patient immediately loses several of his civil rights and for a child who has cancer, MOST civil rights are lost. I'm compelled to tell our story for several reasons. I realized during and after our experience with cancer, that I really didn't know what cancer is, and how inadequate the treatment for this type of cancer truly is, in America. I want to expose the true state of osteosarcoma cancer treatment, and research in America, and change the way our nation is handling this cancer problem.

CANCER Research…Come every April, the fundraising starts… pink ribbons, daffodils, races and walks for THE CURE. I assumed, probably like many American citizens, that scientists in our country are working feverishly night and day to find a cure. Sad to say, IT ISN'T SO! When my daughter was diagnosed, I immediately started to research the condition, and was horrified at what I learned.

1. Osteosarcoma incidence has increased by over 40% in the past 10 years.
2. No one in the research community is interested in this fact.
3. Childhood cancer has overtaken every other illness as the cause of death in children
4. There are no survival statistics for children past five years. The forty year practice where my daughter was treated could only produce ONE ten year survivor of osteosarcoma, and she lived 400 miles away. They tout a 65% success rate for this disease, but it isn't true.
5. Doctors say that they don't know what causes it, but there are convincing smoking guns. The fluoride added to our water causes osteosarcoma in rats. Communities with fluoridated water have higher incidences of osteosarcoma than communities that don't, especially in boys. As children, many of us received tainted polio vaccine (actually 98 million of us). It was contaminated

with a monkey virus called SV40 (more about this in our vaccine section). Our government hid this information from us. Doctors are finding this virus in rare tumors like osteosarcoma, mesothelioma, and certain brain tumors. These children have INHERITED this virus from us, as they have not received tainted polio vaccine. One of the first acts of President George W. Bush was to protect the pharmaceutical companies from lawsuits related to vaccine damage. The executives know what is coming with the revelations of this crime against humanity, and they wanted financial protection. By the way, SV40 is used in cancer research because it is "the perfect little war machine". It causes cancer faster than any other agent at their disposal.

I know these facts are disturbing. It is appalling that we, as Americans, have been deceived by our government for so long, but it is time for it to STOP. Our children are depending upon us to protect them until they can protect themselves. As parents and citizens, it is our duty to take action.

The truly disheartening fact is that this information is so OLD. The government has been undermining its citizens for at least fifty years, maybe longer. Big Business had hi-jacked our government before I was even born. I take part of the responsibility, because as a US citizen I should have taken the time to see what my government was up to. I didn't, and I have paid a heavy price for that neglect. MY goal, for the time I have remaining on this earth, is to challenge these corporations and the government they control, and restore the rights they have stolen from us.

Nixon declared a "WAR ON CANCER" during his administration. This concept gave the misleading impression that our government was serious about solving the cancer problem. Thinking people have suspected for many years that a cure for cancer has been suppressed. The truth is there have been numerous cures for osteosarcoma through the years.

Anyone who has accomplished one of these miracles, has been harassed, murdered, ruined or kept quiet about it. The medical cartel WILL NOT give up the riches they have gotten from the exploitation of the sickest and weakest in our society. THEY are the true cancer in our society, and it is time for radical surgery to eliminate them.

We actually had my daughter's condition under control for four and a half years before she became ill again. My daughter's tumor was very small at the time of diagnosis. We caught it very early, BUT THAT DID NOT MATTER, because cancer is a disease of the blood. The tumor is the end product of that lethal disease. Treating the tumor does not solve the problem. After months of chemotherapy and radical surgery, only 1 CENTIMETER OF TUMOR WAS DESTROYED. We decided to try alternative therapies, as it was obvious that her treatment protocol was not working. Her oncologist threatened to SUE US FOR CUSTODY of our daughter. You know, I waited until I was thirty-one years old to have my daughter. She was the light of my life. I was blessed with the gift of this child, and enjoyed every moment of her time with us. I found it disgusting for her doctor to suggest that I didn't have her welfare at heart and that the GOVERNMENT would be a better parent than the parents she had. I told her doctor (who had been suffering with allergies the entire time she was treating my daughter) that she couldn't even solve her own minor health issues, let alone something as serious as cancer. I told her that I would welcome a lawsuit and custody fight, because the medical staff would have to go to court and PROVE that their treatments were effective. They would have to provide patients they had cured and show that the treatment protocol they prescribed had benefit for my daughter. She walked out of the room and never brought it up again. The LAST THING the child cancer industry wants is to go into a court and prove that what they do has any positive benefit for patients, BECAUSE THEY CAN'T.

We stopped Brett's treatment when the chemo had damaged her liver and started to cause her hemoglobin to DISINTEGRATE. We decided to take her to the Livingston

Foundation Medical Center in San Diego. The research I had done convinced me that the key to defeating cancer was repairing the damage to a person's immune system, that a well functioning immune system does not allow tumors to form. The medical community has known this since the early 1900's. Dr. Livingston, from western Pennsylvania, was a brilliant woman. She was one of the great sorts of doctor who is a rarity in modern medicine. She knew what it meant to be a REAL doctor, not the morally bankrupt technicians in the industry today who pass as doctors. Brett was evaluated at the Livingston Foundation Medical Center with tests hospitals don't do and given vaccines that hospitals can't provide. She was shown how to eat to live with health. She stayed healthy for four years. The Livingston Foundation Medical Center, after 32 years, had to close, because the FDA would not allow them to advertise what a tremendous job they did helping patients with cancer and immune diseases. The reason we took Brett to this clinic was because they had a track record of curing children with sarcomas. I don't know of any business in the world that could survive for thirty- two years without being permitted to advertise. Brett's vaccines were only about $50 a month. I guess that is the major reason that pharmaceutical companies desperately suppress immunotherapy solutions to cancer. They cannot profit from these children and desperately sick adults if this therapy is used. Dr. Livingston had found a remedy for cancer long ago, and she knew she was just one of many who had. Within six months of no vaccines, my daughter Brett had an enormous tumor in her left lung.

    During my research I came across the unique drug called Ukrain that was developed about twenty-five years ago. It basically is a non-toxic chemo. Even after this much time this terrific drug only has orphan drug status in the US for pancreatic cancer. It only adheres to cancer cells and leaves healthy cells alone. When a patient receives it, a patient's hair doesn't fall out, mouth sores the size of quarters do not form, people don't throw up, actually Ukrain enhances the immune system, instead of harming it. It has been tested at our National Cancer Institute and it worked on fifty-seven out of sixty cancer cell lines. It is relatively inexpensive and easy to administer compared to American Chemo. The inventor, Dr. Nowicky has endured endless harassment from the pharmaceutical cartel. I think CARTEL is the appropriate description for these corporations. It is criminal to hold sick patients hostage with their deadly ineffective drugs. I had spoken with many people who used Ukrain for a variety of cancers very successfully. Brett's doctors here informed us there was nothing they could do for her. No surgery, chemo, or radiation could help her. We decided to go to Germany to a clinic that helped children with deadly sarcomas, which had been declared incurable by the American Medical Cartel. The German protocol consisted of Ukrain administered with hyperthermia (another established cancer treatment that is scarce in America), vaccine therapy, and cancer cocktails of nutrients to rebuild the body. After ten days we returned home. Brett was so much improved. She ran through the Frankfurt airport, her tumor markers were coming down and we were filled with hope. I legally brought the Ukrain home with me. There was only one doctor who would administer it to her (it is an IV drug). Her primary care doctor refused, even though it was legal to have it. We were to return to Germany in six weeks for continued treatment. Brett developed a lung infection and had to be rushed to the hospital. She was in intensive care on a breathing tube for two weeks. They wanted to pull her tube and let her die, but we were outraged. Their procedures had landed her in worse shape than when she arrived. We insisted that she be given her Ukrain treatment. We signed papers absolving the hospital and doctors of any responsibility. Brett received the Ukrain three times a week for two weeks and was improved enough to be discharged to go home. The doctors recommended she continue with her Ukrain treatment and it was on her discharge papers. They knew it had to be IV administered. No one would come to our house to give it to her. The home nursing company we used that was part of the hospital refused. They give 2500 patients chemo at home in the Pittsburgh area, but they wouldn't give Brett her life-saving medicine. They said the FDA wouldn't allow it. I contacted the FDA, told them the situation, and they denied that they were in the way. I contacted the State Dept of

Medicine in Pennsylvania, and their legal department said they did not have ONE law on the books preventing the doctors from prescribing Brett her medicine. The simple truth is that her doctors let her die. No one in government would help us. I had to watch my beautiful eighteen year old daughter cry and ask me why no one would help her. It is a heartbreak I would not wish on any parent. After four weeks of no drug therapy Brett's health failed. Her doctors would not give permission for her to fly to Germany. This beautiful and brave girl died in the ICU of the hospital where they refused to give her what she needed to fight. Brett asked me to help her die without pain. I told her I would. She had family with her, but she asked to call the ones who could not be there, to tell them she loved them and to say good bye. She told me not to blame myself, that I had done everything I could to help her. She was a magnificent human being who deserved everything this country could offer, but she was denied. She asked me to let people know the truth. It was her last request and I am going to do everything in my power to do that.

Finally, I want to communicate what I think will be agents for change. DON'T contribute to cancer charities, especially the American Cancer Society. They actively are controlled by the pharmaceutical companies and try to discredit anyone truly working on the cancer problem. Refuse treatment here. It doesn't work, and it is shortening the time you have on this earth. Go to other countries for treatment. Even if you want chemo, they do it better, with less suffering. There are clinics that will address your whole problem; they will work with patients on why they got sick in the first place. Pressure insurance companies to pay for treatments that WORK. They only want to pay for what the pharmaceutical companies want to prescribe. We forced our health insurance carrier to reimburse us for Brett's vaccine treatment. It took awhile, but we got it. I promised Brett I would write a more detailed book to help others with cancer get well. I have to keep my promise, as it is the last thing I can do for her in this world. When I meet her again, I want to be able to say I followed through and her death affected humanity in a positive, life-affirming way.

NOTES

Cancer Cured for Good
By Bill Sardi and Timothy Hubbell
October 2008

It works 100% of the time to eradicate cancer completely, and cancer does not recur even years later. That is how researchers describe the most convincing cancer cure ever announced.

The weekly injection of just 100 billionths of a gram of a harmless glyco-protein (a naturally-produced molecule with a sugar component and a protein component) activates the human immune system and cures cancer for good, according to human studies among breast cancer and colon cancer patients, producing complete remissions lasting 4 and 7 years respectively. This glyco-protein cure is totally without side effect but currently goes unused by cancer doctors.

Normal Gc protein (also called Vitamin-D binding protein), an abundant glyco-protein found in human blood serum, becomes the molecular switch to activate macrophages when it is converted to its active form, called Gc macrophage activating factor (Gc-MAF). Gc protein is normally activated by conversion to Gc-MAF with the help of the B and T cells (bone marrow-made and thymus gland-made white blood cells). But, as researchers explain it themselves, cancer cells secrete an enzyme known as alpha-N-acetylgalactosaminidase (also called Nagalase) that completely blocks conversion of Gc protein to Gc-MAF, preventing tumor-cell killing by the macrophages. This is the way cancer cells escape detection and destruction, by disengaging the human immune system. This also leaves cancer patients prone to infections and many then succumb to pneumonia or other infections.

The once-weekly injection of minute amounts of Gc-MAF, just 100 nanograms (billionths of a gram), activates macrophages and allows the immune system to pursue cancer cells with vigor, sufficient to produce total long-term cures in humans.

Nobuto Yamamoto, director of the Division of Cancer Immunology and Molecular Biology, Socrates Institute for Therapeutic Immunology, Philadelphia, Pennsylvania, says this is *"probably the most potent macrophage activating factor ever discovered."*

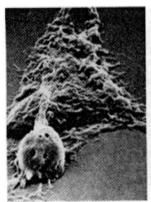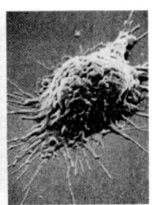

A Macrophage Overcomes And Eats A Cancer Cell.
From The Upjohn Company, The Immune System

Once a sufficient number of activated macrophages are produced, another Gc-MAF injection is not needed for a week because macrophages have a half-life of about six days. After 16-22 weekly doses of Gc-MAF the amount of Nagalase enzyme fell to levels found in healthy people, which serves as evidence tumors have been completely eliminated. The treatment was fool-proof - - - it worked in 100% of 16 breast cancer patients and there were no recurrent tumors over a period of 4 years, says a report in the January

15 issue of the *International Journal of Cancer.* [*International Journal Cancer.*2008 January15; 122(2):461-7]

In another startling follow-up report by Dr. Yamamoto and colleagues, published in the upcoming July issue of Cancer Immunology Immunotherapy, Gc-MAF therapy totally abolished tumors in 8 colon cancer patients who had already undergone surgery but still exhibited circulating cancer cells (metastases). After 32-50 weekly injections, *"all colorectal cancer patients exhibited healthy control levels of the serum Nagalase activity, indicating eradication of metastatic tumor cells,"* said researchers, an effect that lasted 7 years with no indication of cancer recurrence either by enzyme activity or CT scans, said researchers. [*Cancer Immunology, Immunotherapy* Volume 57, Number 7 / July 2008] Published in an early online edition of this journal, this confirming report has received no attention by the new media so far, despite its striking importance.

Gc-MAF treatment for cancer has been agonizingly slow to develop. Dr. Yamamoto first described this immunotherapy in 1993. [*The Journal of Immunology*, 1993 151 (5); 2794-2802]

In a similar animal experiment published in 2003, researchers in Germany, Japan and the United States collaborated to successfully demonstrate that after they had injected macrophage activating factor (Gc-MAF) into tumor-bearing mice, it totally eradicated tumors. [*Neoplasia* 2003 January; 5(1): 32-40]

In 1997 Dr. Yamamoto injected GcMAF protein into tumor-bearing mice, with the same startling results. A single enzyme injection doubled the survival of these mice and just four enzyme injections increased survival by 6-fold. [*Cancer Research* 1997 Jun 1; 57(11):2187-92]

In 1996 Dr. Yamamoto reported that all 52 cancer patients he had studied carried elevated blood plasma levels of the immune inactivating alpha-N-acetylgalactosaminidase enzyme (Nagalase), whereas healthy humans had very low levels of this enzyme. [*Cancer Research* 1996 Jun 15; 56(12):2827-31]

In the early 1990s, Dr. Yamamoto first described how the human immune system is disengaged by enzymes secreted from cancer cells, even filing a patent on the proposed therapy. [US Patent 5326749, July 1994; *Cancer Research* 1996 June 15; 56: 2827-31]

Activated Gc protein has been used in humans at much higher doses without side effect. This Gc macrophage activating factor (Gc-MAF) has been shown to be effective against a variety of cancers including breast, prostate, stomach, liver, lung, uterus, ovary, brain, skin, head/neck cancer, and leukemia.

Although GcMAF is also called Vitamin-D binding protein, the activation of macrophages does not require Vitamin D.

It cannot be said the Gc-MAF cancer cure has gone unheralded. Reuters News covered this developing story in January. But the news story still did not receive top billing nor did it fully elucidate the importance of the discovery, actually made years ago, that the human body is capable of abolishing cancer once its immune system is properly activated.

GcMAF is a naturally made molecule and is not patentable, though its manufacturing process is patent protected. There is no evidence of any current effort to commercialize this therapy or put it into practice. Should such an effective treatment for cancer come into common practice, the income stream from health-insurance plans for every oncology office and cancer center in the world Would likely be reduced to the point of financial insolvency and hundreds of thousands of jobs would be eliminated.

The National Cancer Institute estimates cancer care in the U.S. costs ~$72 billion annually (2004). Furthermore, about $55 billion of cancer drugs are used annually, none which have not significantly improved survival rates throughout the history of their use. If a typical cancer patient had to undergo

30 GcMAF injections at a cost of $150 per injection, that would cost ~$4500, not counting doctor's office visits and follow-up testing. For comparison, gene-targeted cancer drugs range from $13,000 to $100,000 in cost per year and produce only marginal improvements in survival (weeks to months). [*Targeted Oncology* 2007 April, 2 (2); 113-19]

Up to this point, the National Cancer Institute is totally silent on this discovery and there is no evidence the cancer care industry plans to quickly mobilize to use this otherwise harmless treatment.

Addendum: Sadly, the treatment you have just read about is not available anywhere. Its inventor is attempting to patent a version of it to profiteer off of it even though there is no need to improve upon the GcMAF molecule - - it worked without failure to completely cure four different types of cancer with no long-term remissions and without side effect. While GcMAF is produced by every healthy adult, there are no centers available to extract it from blood samples and inject it into patients with malignancies. Hopefully, someday, doctors will write protocols to do this and submit them to institutional review boards so GcMAF treatment can be performed on an experimental basis. GcMAF is a naturally-made molecule that cannot be patented. This article was written to reveal that there are proven cancer cures that go unused. Of interest, not one oncologist has requested information about GcMAF since this article was written, while I have been barraged with inquires from cancer patients, their families and some interested physicians who are not cancer doctors. -Bill Sardi

Based in Southern California, Bill Sardi is a notedand well-known author, lecturer, speaker, and health researcher, with numerous books and articles to his credit. He can be reached at BSardi@aol.com. Timothy Hubbell, a biochemist from

Cincinnati, first called attention to this discovery and provided consultation on the biochemistry.

Help NHF get the word out about GcMAF and other proven cures for cancer that are being ignored. Learn how NHF is the leading health freedom organization, for example, battling for your right to maintain access to dietary supplements without restrictions imposed by quasi-governing bodies like CODEX and our other missions. Search the NHF website for more helpful information and become a member by clicking here.

REBATE

Please fill out this form and receive a $3.00 rebate on your purchase.

Name: _____

Address: _____
_____

Email: _____ Phone: _____

Store Name: _____ Online Store: _____

Please attach original receipt of purchase.

Comments about the book: _____
_____
_____
_____

Mail to: Friends of the Planet
          1000 Thorn Run Rd.
          Pittsburgh, Pa 15108
Email: friends-of-the-planet@hotmail.com
Phone: 412.741.7471

LaVergne, TN USA
19 January 2011
213095LV00009B/69/P